INTEGRAL HEALING

Lynne D. Feldman

Integral Publishers

Tucson, Arizona 85712

© 2014 Integral Publishers

Integral Publishers
1418 N. Jefferson Ave.
Tucson AZ 85712
831 333-9200

ISBN: 978-0-9904419-0-8

Covver design by Jeannie Carlisle

To Erica and Adam, my beloveds

For a Radiant Star

I know not what to do
Yet giddy with instinct
Throw myself out,
Caught by a current unseen,
Swoop low, glide high, dive
Into surrender.

A chrysalis stands now empty,
Drying in the sun,
Constraints forgotten by the life once served.

One day, perhaps, a child will come,
Will ask its mother,
"What strange creature one day lived
In such a tiny home?"

– Treya Wilber, 1974,
as quoted in *Grace and Grit*

TABLE OF CONTENTS

FOREWORD

Ken Wilber

Lynne Feldman has written a book specifically for "patients," those with an identified medical illness – and those for whom traditional medical treatments just don't cover nearly enough territory to make them feel confident of any real cure. Instead, using a revolutionary new framework called Integral Theory – which is a fully comprehensive "map" of the human condition, drawing on Western and Eastern, scientifc and spiritual and moral and aesthetic methods – she has crafted an approach to any illness that literally touches all the bases – in both cause and cure – and thus has the highest chance of actually affecting any disease process in a truly healing and curative fashion. When a well-respected physician just released evidence that chemotherapy only works on 1 in 10 patients, how on earth can anybody trust using only orthodox Western medical models? Yet in other areas – say, cataract disease, where Western surgery cures 95% of patients – why on earth would you want to forgo Western treatment altogether and just rely on, say, meditation?

What is needed is a way to put all of these treatments together into a single framework, then use that overall framework to point the way to which treatments are likely to work, and which treatments are likely to fail, and then draw together all the positive treatments into a truly comprehensive approach to healing. Using Integral Theory, this is what Lynne managed to do, and anyone suffering from any sort of illness can benefit enormously from applying the methods of Integral Healing to whatever illness they are suffering from.

How does this approach work? Well, Integral Theory itself is a "map" or "framework" drawn from examining literally all the major maps of the human psyche and being from the significant cultures around the world (premodern, modern, and postmodern), and – using each map to fill in any gaps in the others – arrived at a truly all-inclusive map of the human being, the first of its type anywhere in the world. The point is that if you want a comprehensive or inclusive approach to any issue – educational, political, legal, medical, historical, therapeutic, artistic, spiritual, etc. – you simply use this Framework and make sure all of its elements are addressed, thus being asssured of covering all the really important bases. The Framework itself has five major elements, called "quadrants," "levels," "lines," "states," and "types." To show how it works, I'll use the quadrants.

Integral Theory concluded – after looking at all the previous cross-cultural maps of the human being (and of reality itself) – that every phenomenon can be looked at from four major perspectives: the inside and the outside in the individual and the collective. This gives four major dimensions: 1) the inside of the individual (the subjective quadrant, the 1st-person singular, the "I" space, accessed by introspection or "looking within"); 2) the outside of the individual (the objective quadrant, the 3rd-person singular, a distanced or objective "scientific" view of things); 3) the inside of the collective or group (the intersubjective quadrant, a 2nd-person "you" and 1st-person plural "we," the shared values, ethics, roles, and rules of a particular group, its culture; and 4) the outside of the collective (the interobjective quadrant, 3rd-person plural, or how the group looks from the outside in an objective stance, the shared structures, systems, or institutions of the group, the social aspect – including various educational systems, legal systems, environmental systems, eco-systems, etc.).

Now, there are models of the causes and cures of illness that focus on each of those quadrants, and confine their attention to just that quadrant. The standard Western, orthodox, establishment medical system looks only at quadrant #2, the objective organism as approached by modern science. And it treats only the objective organism (with surgery, radiation, medication, chemotherapy, etc.) and believes the cause of the illness comes solely from that quadrant. Many spiritual systems, on the other hand, look only at quadrant

#1, the subjective sphere, the seat of consciousness, the "I," the True Self, and Spirit, and maintains that if you are in touch with that, you will be healed (and becoming out of touch with that is what caused your illness in the first place). The biosocial approach to medicine looks at quadrant #4, the relationship between the organism and its ecological environment, and sees the cause of illness as a mismatch in this sphere, with environmental toxins, environmental stress, and ecological despoliation causing correlative illnesses in the organisms in that ecological system (humans included). The relational approach to medicine looks at quadrant #3, the interpersonal relationship sphere, and sees stress and imbalances in that sphere – with one›s spouse, work-related stress and problems with one›s boss, parental stress and child-rearing issues, or issues with one's parents as one was being raised oneself – as the ultimate cause (and cure) of illness.

Which is right? According to Integral Theory, all of them – because every phenomenon has all four quadrants. More precisely, every illness has some degree of causative factors from all four quadrants. This intuitively makes sense, because as you go around the quadrants, you can understand how problems in that area could indeed cause illness. The problem is, no medical model anywhere includes all four – except the Integral model. Since every illness has some degree of causal factors in every quadrant, that means the cure for every illness needs to address problems in all four areas. But this is something no medical model at all will tell you. This is something you have to figure out yourself, and then look at the various types of cures available in each quadrant (and there are many!), and then put together a specific healing program that addresses the specific dysfunctions you have in each quadrant, and treats all of them together. Only in that way will you be assured of "covering all the bases" – only in that way will be you dealing with all of the causes of your illness – and therefore giving yourself the best possible chance of recovery.

This is what Lynne's book will help you do. She goes through each of the five elements of the Integral Map and shows how each can affect your health or illness, and the types of treatments she sought in each of them, putting together a fully Integral approach to her own healing.

One of the things I have found fascinating as I put together the Integral Framework is how few of its components most people have even heard of, even though all of them possess each and every one of these components, and each one is fully operating in them right now. Many people began intuiting some of these other factors (like the quadrants) when they began to demand alternative and complementary approaches to modern medicine. Many began to find real value in addressing quadrant #1 – the subjective "I" domain – as they began exploring the very positive effects of visualization, affirmation, and meditation on their illness. They also began demanding that their doctors make these treatments available to them (reluctantly, and slowly, the medical establishment began to address at least a few of these items, and most medical schools now have departments of complementary medicine, although still not taken very seriously by "real" doctors, even though empirical evidence continues to accumulate as to their very real effectiveness – meditation, for example, is consistently shown to be more effective in pain management than morphine). But rarely do alternative approaches take into account "relationship" factors – either subjectively/culturally (quadrant #4) or objectively/socially (quadrant #3). But there, too, evidence continues to accumulate (e.g., job-related stress depressing the immune system in quadrant #3, or environmental toxins such as asbestos or radon in quadrant #4). Doesn't it just make sense to admit that all four quadrants have a role to play in both the cause and the cure of illness? Failure to take all four into account simply means you are leaving huge gaps in your diagnosis and treatment protocols, and are thus all that less likely to obtain a genuine cure.

This is the promise and the hope of a truly Integral approach to medicine – both as a physician practitioner, a nurse, and the patients themselves. Adding all five factors together gives us, for the first time in history, a truly comprehensive framework through which to approach human suffering and sickness – and its treatment and hopefully cure. This approach is not awaiting some science fiction future – it is available right now, ready to be put into operation by anyone who is willing to take a modest amount of time to learn its essentials. This is what Lynne herself did, and you will see her unpack and apply each of the major Integral elements to seeing, understanding, and treating all the important causative factors in her very serious illness – and, for now, "winning" that battle. Yet, from another angle, she has permanently won this "contest," because winning can be defined not as beating a physical illness in the exterior individual sphere, but discovering one›s True Self – Spirit itself – in the individual interior realm (the Kingdom of Heaven that is found "within") and since this is definitely a part of the Integral approach, this is a discovery that Lynne most definitely made, a discovery good for all eternity.

I invite you to follow Lynne in her discovery of an Integral Approach to diagnosis, understanding, and treatment, including the spiritual dimension of one's True Self, unborn and undying. The next time you – or anybody you know and care about – becomes ill, you'll be very glad you did, because you'll have many more areas through which to look for possible causes, and many more actions you will be able to take to help effect a cure. No more will you have to reduce "body, mind, and Spirit in self, culture, and nature" to just a physical body with physical treatments, but instead you will be able to span the entire spectrum of consciousness in all major realms of being for both the causes and the cures. An incredible sense of abundance and fulfillment will replace the normal deprivation and scarcity, and you will have the sense, finally, of having come Home.

— Denver, Colorado, Winter 2013

ACKNOWLEDGMENTS

I am grateful to my dear friends, colleagues, and family who gave me the strength and courage to write this book about my complex life and its physical, mental, psychological, and spiritual challenges. Nomi Naeem and Renate Kierey gave me valuable feedback on the memoir portion and persuaded me that the project had merit. I cannot thank my dear and brilliant friend Robin Reinach enough for standing by me and offering her talented insights. I had the finest duo of professional editors: Jacob Miller prodded and supported me into remembering repressed material from my life. He taught me how to switch from my normal terse legal writing style into one that could render scenes from memory that added poignancy to my story. Second, I am indebted to the tender ministrations of Lynwood Lord who helped me express the bounty offered by the Integral model to the field of healthcare. My two guides/therapists/spiritual teachers Lorraine Antine and Patricia Kay continue to help me weave the strands of my life together into a healthier whole, and I am eternally grateful for their support.

My small but tightly knit family earns the highest praise for holding me, sometimes physically, others by cheerleading, and sometimes by their mere presence as I went through the ordeal of two separate cancers and three very serious surgeries along with five months of chemotherapy. This book contains episodes from my stepdaughter's life when she was young and ill. All of these behaviors and symptoms lapsed beginning in her 20s. Now as a grown woman she shines with health of mind and spirit as a mother, wife, daughter, and nurse. It was she who cared for me after my mastectomy with an open heart and loving kindness. I am so proud to call her my daughter today. She has conquered her own difficult past in her own unique way. But to protect her confidentiality, I have changed her name as well as those of many others in the book.

Daughter Erica Leigh and son-in-law Simon believed in my strength and return of good health, and gave me boundless love during and after my illnesses. Little grandson Adam Nathan gave me his presence in my arms when I needed a baby to hold to give me warmth and tenderness.

My dear husband Rick has been the best cheerleader anyone with a serious illness could have. He was a faithful chauffeur, companion, chef, masseur, and love during my illness, and a source of fun and security during all of our forty-two years together.

I owe boundless gratitude to Ken Wilber, who shared his beloved wife Treya's brave battle with breast cancer and who wove her journals and his philosophy into *Grace and Grit*. I owe a great deal to this book and to his groundbreaking thought. I also owe him a great debt for being the person who "saw" me so that I could see myself and my Original Face.

Upper Saddle
River, New Jersey
Winter, 2013

A NOTE TO THE READERS

This book is part memoir and part user's guide as I offer a new approach to healing and flourishing in the face of serious illness, be it a personal challenge, a loved one's, or a client's. It represents a new approach called *Integral Healing*, and it takes the patient, loved one, or healer from initial diagnosis through a transformative journey.

When I was suddenly faced with a cascade of emotional and physical challenges associated with cancer diagnoses, several of them life threatening, I was fortunate to have a comprehensive framework to make sense of all the upheaval. My task over those frightening months was to put the pieces together into an integrated whole. Wilber's articulation of Integral Theory is often referred to as the AQAL (pronounced "*ah*-kwal") model. I had been searching for such a framework all of my adult life. When serious illnesses struck, I used the model to piece together a customized and customizable healing program.

There are countless works now available for the public to learn the basics of Integral Theory, but this book is geared to be accessible to anyone (Those interested in learning about Integral Theory in depth have but to look up Wilber's works). I applied its components and practices to form the structure of the book and upon which to base an Integral Healing Practice. I then used them to guide me on my own continuing healing journey, and I offer it to be adopted and adapted to your own personal challenges.

The series of repeatable phases I discovered within the healing cycle has been adapted from Lewis Richmond's work on aging which runs from *lightning strikes*, to *coming to terms*, to *adaptation*, to *appreciation*. Digging deeply into these phases each time a crisis hit, I was able to approach my journey with more focused consciousness, and to metabolize the crises more quickly. Change is part of existence, and during illness these changes can occur frequently. To be able to cycle from panic to stability to bliss is a rare gift, and one that the Integral framework makes possible.

None of us can chart the arc of our lives; some of us will need healing once, some many times. Ultimately our choice comes down to how well we can transform that which we can, breath by breath, moment by moment, day by day. And that brings us to ultimate fulfillment. My arc began with difficulty. It would be up to me to change its trajectory.

I have lived a challenging and intense life since before I was born. My mother had pre-eclampsia during her pregnancy with me, and "we" spent the last month prior to my birth in the hospital in an attempt to lower her high blood pressure.

Physical assaults and psychological traumas followed me throughout my life. I reasoned I had suffered enough over the span of many decades that my immune system had been sensitized to recognize and fight against the most diabolical of maladies, cancer, but the opposite proved to be true. The serial distresses of my life weakened my immune system and set up significant internal chaos so that I wound up with a run of illnesses commencing in fall 2010. Against my lifetime belief that I was destined to be a victim of some sad fate, being a cancer victim spurred me to seek a different mindset and to construct a healing path that is based on what is known as Integral Life Practice. It called me to revisit my earlier traumas and begin to resolve them. How else was I to create a healthy ecology within which to nurture my healing? With this call to do as deep a dive as possible, I sought to construct my unique version of an Integral Healing Program to join the other modules presented in what is called an Integral Life Practice. So far it has worked, sometimes against significant medical and psychological odds.

I have not written about any person in this book with the intention, either express or unintended, of disparaging them. The integral model correctly explains that we can "see" only our individual subjective perspectives on events in our lives. Others will have their own subjective perspectives on the same occurrences. I have dealt with my perspective not as the absolute truth of the matter, but as to how it affected me psychologically and physically.

I humbly offer this book as a journey by one woman who faced considerable challenges, as well as a guidebook for anyone who must confront serious illness.

PART 1

LIGHTNING STRIKES

CHAPTER ONE

It Begins

Dr. Woodward wasn't smiling. Her streaked blond hair fell loose to her shoulders; she sat erect behind her desk at the modern Heights Breast Cancer Center, which stood at the top of a rolling hill near a hospital. I took the chair across from her. It was September 2010, the day after my return from a spiritual retreat in Sedona, Arizona. I was centered, calm, and inspired, ready for anything. The nurse silently folded herself into a seat beside mine.

"Why aren't you smiling?" I tried to tease Dr. Woodward who looked inordinately serious.

"I never smile when I have to give bad news."

I was puzzled, but not alarmed. Hadn't Dr. Woodward encouraged me to attend the retreat? Prior to my departure she told me she felt strongly that my needle biopsy wouldn't show any sign of cancer.

"You have invasive breast cancer." Dr. Woodward's tone was deadpan. Her face was blank.

I felt as though I had just been struck by lightning. I tried to breathe, but my lungs wouldn't respond to mental commands. Then I began to shake inside. My organs felt as though they whipsawed from front to back in a staccato rhythm until I began to feel faint. No sound emanated from my mouth, but mentally I was very busy commenting on this unexpected result.

Not fair! Not fair! I've had too much bad news already!

"Are you OK?" the nurse gently inquired as she saw my body quake. At my earlier appointment she and I chatted humorously together, but today I wanted to scream at her.

"Do I *look* OK?" I exclaimed when my lungs finally came back online. It was a rare burst of public anger for me. I sucked in enough air to begin spitting out my frustration and rage. But the satisfaction of exploding was short lived. Defeat descended on my shoulders like an invisible cape, and overwhelming fear twisted my gut.

"Am I going to die?" I could barely rasp out the question.

"Lynne, you have run-of-the-mill breast cancer. Just like 80% of women with cancer."

"Run-of-the-mill" for who? In Dr. Woodward's normal workday, perhaps, but not for me. What good was it to know she encountered this type of cancer in so many women in her work? This was *me* and *my* diagnosis. What is the "normal" response to finding out you have breast cancer, anyhow?

The doctor's reasonable tone of voice made me feel stone cold. A hard kind of anger filled my chest. I felt a ragged desire to flee. Instead, I pulled my chair closer to Dr. Woodward's desk, and tried to focus out of the fog that had settled on me. She began to explain the results of my needle biopsy. There seemed to be three entities in the room: Dr. Woodward, who was clearly trying to share important information with me; myself, barely aware of my own feelings or of the content of our conversation; and the cancer that was present in the room, in her words, in my fear, and in my breast.

Sitting in the doctor's office, listening to her explain the cancer growing in my body, I ricocheted between numbness and fury. While my physical self sat mute and listless, Dr. Woodward described "my" cancer without realizing she was giving me too much technological information. My mind heard the words but my emotions prevented me from processing them. Through a numb haze, I heard her say that "my" cancer "was no longer contained within the left breast's milk duct, but has invaded your normal breast tissue and is still aggressive and on the move.

"My" type of invasive cancer. Could there be a more unwanted and unwelcome pronoun?

The doctor sketched some notes and a picture of a breast on construction paper.

"Lynne, here's what the pathology report showed from the needle biopsy. You have infiltrating, moderately differentiated ductal carcinoma, Grade 2. This infiltrating carcinoma is present in 11 foci up to 3 millimeters. The good news is that there doesn't seem to be any evidence of lymph node invasion."

The doctor continued explaining treatment scenarios that my mind couldn't grasp. How would I make decisions about treatment when I had no idea what her words meant?

"You will either have a lumpectomy or a mastectomy."

"Lumpectomy"? "Mastectomy"? I knew little about either of these terms. I knew I'd hit the internet as soon as I got home to learn more. My research would lead me into the foreign land of oncology, a place where strangers held the key to medicines and methods that would decide whether I lived or died. "Cancer-ese" was a foreign language I hadn't yet learned to decipher.

I hated the doctor's voice, her streaked blond hair, and the desk that separated her from me. I hated the nurse, still sitting at my side, yet I wished she would hold my hand.

Dr. Woodward continued talking. "Now, we're going to have to do several more tests before we know how to treat you locally, regionally, or systemically, or all of them."

My mind raced and stumbled on some basic questions. Why had my cells go awry? Why hadn't the doctors and nurses discovered the cancer when they examined me before? Was it a good sign that they couldn't feel the cancer, and did it mean the tumor must be small? Or was it a bad omen because it was so slippery? My mind fell into magical thinking, refusing to process medical information, grasping at straws of superstition instead.

Dr. Woodward hadn't stopped speaking and I managed to pick up on phrases. "Once the tests show us more about your cancer, then we can consider whether to do a lumpectomy, which I think you qualify for, or a mastectomy with or without reconstruction, with chemotherapy and perhaps radiation."

My focus vanished at the word "chemotherapy."

This isn't happening... I'm not in this situation, a voice in my mind repeated like a mantra.

Dr. Woodward may have thought she was being neutral in her demeanor about the treatment possibilities for my "run-of-the-mill cancer." But her "neutral and professional" tone sounded apocalyptic to me. I wanted to throw her chart across the room. Instead, I sat compliantly across the desk until our appointment concluded. As I let the dreaded words that I had cancer continue to flow over me, I lost my inner locus of control and felt powerless. I'd been thrust onto the threshold of an alien place.

With all the passionate innocence of the child I had once been, I wanted Dr. Woodward to promise me that I would have no pain and I wouldn't need chemotherapy. She couldn't, and she didn't. I also desperately wanted to believe Dr. Woodward's reassurances, just as much as I wanted to believe Aunt Ann when she prayed over my mother and me when we got sick.

Aunt Ann was my father's sister. She had left our Jewish faith to become a Christian Scientist and visited often when my mother and I had our routine bouts of asthmatic bronchitis. Ann prayed fervently over us, certain her bible could trump respiratory infections. She made me repeat the affirmation, "The Lord loves me, and I won't get sick." I did, faithfully. But then I felt guilty whenever I did get sick, which was often. Hadn't I prayed hard enough? Didn't the Lord love me enough?

I wanted Dr. Woodward to be an effective version of Aunt Ann. If only the good doctor could assure me that I'd be well, that I would not suffer. I wanted her to tell me what demonic outside force had entered my body. How could my loyal cells have turned rogue? I wanted—at the very least—Dr. Woodward's assurances there were only a few of these rogue cells, and modern medicine would be able to rid my body of the turncoats.

Still half-listening to her explanations, I morphed into a new, compound identity: "cancer victim." Suddenly I bore the label of a woman with cancer; I became the victim of a disease. My body had turned against me and thrust ugliness on me.

My new and deformed self-sense felt odd. How could I be both tightly wound into a small mass and at the same time shattered into random pieces like a Jackson Pollack painting? This odd sensation came from the coiled pressure of the unknown, and the explosion of what I held as "me." What should I do tomorrow? Who cared, now that I stepped into this vast void? "I" had planned for tomorrow's schedule, but it no longer counted. What tomorrow and which identity was I to connect myself to now? The innate, interior patterns of my life had vanished.

I observed a woman walking past Dr. Woodward's door. Looking to be in her thirties, she had swung the doors open and exited from the dreaded chemotherapy room, soothingly labeled the "Infusion Suite." She was wearing a smart little cloche hat, and I wondered if it hid a bald head or whether she still had hair. Her perspective of her condition must be far different than mine. I thought how unfair it must seem to her to have breast cancer at such a young age. She might be married and a mother or contemplating having children, I mused. Thank God I was 65 and well past the age of thinking of having more children. What if she were dating, and dealing with a bald head and perhaps only one breast? What about her self-image as a sexual being? Many cancer treatments plunge women directly into menopause. Would that be her fate?

In that moment I realized that the lightning strike effect I had just experienced must coincide with the stage of maturation of an individual's consciousness. That is, the impact of her diagnosis would depend on the extent to which the young woman was aware, and how she viewed the world. A young woman would have an entirely different perspective on what she was going through than an older woman like me. So would her perspectives on her yesterdays, todays, and tomorrows. I watched her head toward the elevator and lost sight of her.

I got up and went out to the waiting room where I took out my cell phone and called my husband, Rick.

"The news isn't good, hon," I said.

"What are you saying? What does that mean?" His voice was scratchy and near panic.

"The test came back positive. I have invasive breast cancer."

He began to cry.

I returned briefly to the doctor's office to say goodbye to Dr. Woodward and her nurse. I assured her that I'd have more tests to confirm the extent of the cancer. Robotically I walked out of Heights Cancer Center, and passed the beautiful, tasteful, and softly appointed treatment rooms, obviously meant to soothe the most frazzled patient. That would be me. It wasn't working.

You don't fool me, I thought as I glared into the lobby. I exited into the parking lot searching for my car. Finding it after a short hunt, bitter thoughts speared me as I opened the car door. I never asked, "Why me?" *Of course* it was me. I had read enough articles on how breast cancer can take years to develop. It actually made sense that I would have cancer. The series of toxic emotional episodes I was called to metabolize throughout my life had finally manifested into something deadly. The shitty things in my life just kept coming, didn't they? I jerked the transmission into reverse and gunned the car out of the slot. I drove to the highway on-ramp with a vice-like grip on the wheel and scattered consciousness. I almost rammed into a silver Mercedes, where the driver honked and screamed at me until I swerved back into my proper lane.

I had twenty minutes of driving time getting home to engage in perplexed reverie. *Wasn't I the poster-girl of victimization? Hadn't my mother's family taught me that they were inflicted with what my mother called "the curse of the Greenbergs"? This cancer diagnosis was just another bad luck part of my life.*

The phone rang the second I entered the empty house. It was Rick. "Hon, listen, I'm gonna get you the best doctors around, so don't lose hope."

"I love you," I responded with a whisper. I held onto his words even though I could tell that his usual alpha-male, self-assured personality had been replaced with fear. But his words still gave me the strength to go to my office. I left the safe haven of the kitchen, the very heart of my home, and climbed the stairs. I went immediately to my computer, and let the professional researcher in me take over while I stayed numb. The persona of the professional researcher separated me from the persona of the frightened child who thought she would die of cancer. This professional discovered that every year, nearly 250,000 women learn they have invasive breast cancer. About 58,000 more are diagnosed with early stages of the disease. And approximately 40,000 of us will die (Arun et al., 2010).

What would this journey through invasive breast cancer be like? The only experience I had was secondhand from reading integral philosopher and author Ken Wilber's poignant story of his beloved wife Treya's unsuccessful five-year battle with breast cancer in *Grace and Grit.* Other than that, I had no idea what a cancer diagnosis involved. I had to muster the courage to re-read Wilber's book that first week, and found a resonant chord:

> Strange things happen to the mind when catastrophe strikes. It felt like the universe turned into a thin paper tissue, and then someone simply tore the tissue in half right in front of my eyes....A tremendous strength descended on me, the strength of being totally jolted and totally stupefied....As Samuel Johnson drily commented, the prospect of death marvelously concentrates the mind. (Wilber, 2000, p. 47)

Earlier, Wilber recounts part of Treya's feelings of shock and anger at her diagnosis:

> This is real. This is happening to me. I lie in bed rigid with shock and disbelief as the world lies quiet around me....I have cancer. I have breast cancer. I believe this is true and, at the same time, I do not believe it; I cannot let it in....
>
> CANCER. CANCER. CANCER. This cannot be undone, this cannot be erased. CANCER. A cloud of voices, images, ideas, fears, stories, photographs, advertisements, articles, movies, television shows arises around me, vague, shapeless, but dense, ominous. These are the stories my culture has collected around this thing, 'the big C.' (*Ibid*, pp. 39-40)

Treya's comment about stories from her culture stayed with me personally as I thought about my own family and their phobias about illness. But Wilber makes a significant distinction between the concepts of "illness" and of "sickness." "Illness" is the actual disease process facing me, be it a broken bone or a malignant tumor. It has medical and scientific dimensions, and is more or less value-free—a typical external entity of my physical system. I was plenty familiar with illness, including a history of asthmatic-bronchitis and multiple cases of pneumonia. My daughter Erica had been routinely hospitalized with asthma since infancy, and my stepdaughter Melissa, Rick's daughter from his first marriage, had been born with neurofibromatosis. Rick himself had been hospitalized for a month in 1978 with a serious heart infection and more recently, in 1999, had serious heart surgery to repair a valve and an aortic aneurism. My little family had certainly experienced "illness."

"Sickness," on the other hand, is how my culture—my family, friends, community, and nation—judged me while having that illness, with all the fears, hopes, myths, stories, and values that accompany that judgment. If the culture treats a particular illness with compassion and enlightened understanding, argues Wilber, then sickness can be seen as a challenge, a healing crisis and opportunity. But what about the opposite situation? I recalled the early days of AIDS, when socially conservative religious people deemed it a punishment for biblically prohibited behavior. The poor homosexuals afflicted with AIDS in the 1980s suffered not only from a horrid disease, but from their culture's condemnation. Pre-modern cultures might heal or condemn a community member to die if he shares their mythic beliefs.

With this distinction before me, I read as many recent publications on the "breast cancer enterprise" as I could find. I looked closely at the cultural aspects associated with having breast cancer. I spent time examining myself for any toxic cultural beliefs, both ignorantly negative and naively optimistic.

I did a self evaluation. How was I reacting emotionally as well as intellectually to my diagnosis? I certainly couldn't figure out what was going to happen to me. Cancer was either going to kill me or it wasn't. It felt that simple to me. But with time to process this *lightning strike*, I realized I had something reliable to cling to. I didn't have to settle for irrational thought patterns handed down to me by my mother's family.

Being a spiritually active person, I wanted to see how my new physical situation might connect with my body, mind, and spirit.

What was I feeling in the deepest part of my heart? Was I thinking I would die? Did I really believe a part or aspect of me would live on after my death? Did I have the strength to stop any habits that contributed to my suffering? Did I have the capacity to transform and replace those habits? Did I truly believe that I could be at peace and express myself with love at a challenging time like this?

Considering these ultimate issues led me to connect with what I call the *Ground of Being*, or the divine aspect of my life as a human being. That connection, if I could keep it strong and constant, gave me a glimmer of hope. I could find some nuanced understanding that would free me from a simple choice of life or death.

Still feeling disoriented as I sat in front of my computer that first night looking up breast cancer mortality statistics, I started focusing on my awareness of being in human form. It was difficult since I felt alien to myself at that moment. I was, truly, diseased and dis-eased by the day's catastrophic findings.

I also had to factor in the overwhelming psychological and spiritual damage I'd incurred over my lifetime. By now I had received a diagnosis of Generalized Anxiety, and I felt I had earned it the hard way. The multiple *lightning strikes* I had experienced affected my psyche, my organs, my memory, and my very cells.

I began teaching myself Integral Theory in 1982, and felt it offered enough information and direction to figure out a plan of action for my upcoming cancer battle. The Integral model permitted me to look at as many comprehensive, inclusive, non-marginalizing, and embracing approaches to all of the possible eventualities I might face. None need be excluded. It also encompassed areas of human knowledge that I would need to cope during this battle for my life. I'd have to do reparative work on my negative and injured self-esteem through deep psychological processes and self-inquiry; I'd have to select the healthiest foods, body practices, and medical interventions of all sorts to deal with the disease; I'd want to reconnect with my support system by both giving and receiving love; and I'd investigate the finest protocols known to date for treating "my" breast cancer.

From Wilber's earliest books to his most recent writings, I had become aware of what constituted my "worldview." I had to identify any constricted beliefs, or what Wilber deemed a *pre-rational level* of understanding. This level of consciousness is akin to my mother's belief in the existence of a "Greenberg curse" on our family, or indigenous peoples' belief in ghosts or spirits from their ancestors.

How I saw the world that first night was a more modern and rational awareness of what life encompasses. A modern, *rational level* of awareness is most commonly associated with science and a belief in the concrete nature of matter. This led to a belief that God was a watchmaker who set the world ticking and then left it to operate scientifically and mechanistically. My doctors subscribed to the rational part of the world's functioning and most likely did not go beyond what the concrete world had to offer them.

There is also an expansive embrace of life akin to what the great spiritual masters see during their meditations and spiritual practices. The *trans-rational*, or postmodern, view of existence allows for the prospect of states of consciousness that embrace the highest possibilities of human potential. I thought of my mother's phenomenal creative abilities and her actions under self-hypnosis. Returning to my dining room, I scanned the seven huge oil paintings she had completed over her lifetime that hung there. The oils gushed with the vibrancy of nature, with birds, butterflies, and different species of summer flowers.

My considerations of what medical options fit into the three categories of pre-rational, rational, and trans-rational began in fits and starts that night. But over time I integrated more and more of what I needed throughout my journey with cancer. My pre-rational thoughts first led me down the "cancer victim" path of ill fate, which my mother had taught me was destiny.

Cancer Victim

My next assignment was to Google "cancer victim," which yielded 78 million sources. I also located 2,600 works on Amazon's book list using the same search term. I had gone through my life as a professional victim. The moniker was imprinted deep within my DNA. Now I had one more tagline to add as a cancer victim. I feared this compound term might come to define me. I knew from victimology theories by experts such as Ann Wolpert Burgess and Cheryl Regehr that my turbulent background left me at risk for a host of adverse psychological consequences, from depression to suicidal ideation.

I next unearthed the origins of the words that had come to define me. These etymology explorations yielded the history of terms and suffused them with emotions and ancient energy. I found that the word "victim" came from the late 15th century and tied in with the idea of scapegoating. A victim is any living creature killed as a sacrifice to a power or entity considered supernatural by the one doing the offering (Online Etymology Dictionary). I found all of these connotations objectionable. The idea of myself on the altar of some operating room ready to be sacrificed in a holy ritual left me completely unnerved.

Yet somehow the term "cancer victim" seemed like a misnomer. I needed to separate out the victim idea from the sickness and the illness. A victim is generally viewed as someone with responsibility for his own limiting beliefs, and who has settled into becoming a victim to his innermost ideation. If I identified as a cancer victim, I would have abdicated my responsibility to jettison the idea that I was a victim. Culturally we tend to permit others to dictate how we feel, what we think, and what label we permit to be hung around our neck. I'd have to be careful when I called my friends and told them of the diagnosis; I didn't want them to consider me as a victim.

That night I had to first call my daughter and inform her. The rest and centering I had achieved during my retreat in Sedona had vanished during the hour spent at Heights Cancer Center receiving my diagnosis. I was in some new dimension of time and place when I got home that night. Erica answered the call with happy news.

"Guess what, Eema [Hebrew for mother]?"

"Sweetie, I have some news too..."

"No, me first! I'm starting shots so that I can get pregnant, Eema! We're going to have a baby!" She was giggling furiously at this news, and who could blame her? She had married the man of her dreams, they had bought a house that they adored a mile away from us, and they both had solid jobs they enjoyed.

"Oh...Sweetheart...how marvelous."

She heard my dead tone to her happy news and abruptly changed from giggling to concerned adult. "What happened? What did they tell you?"

"I have breast cancer, hon…"

"Ohmygodno!" she screamed.

"…but it really isn't as bad as it sounds. Eighty percent of women who have breast cancer have my kind, and I'm not going to die, so it's a bad break, but we'll deal with it." I was not about to upset my daughter, and returned to my typical guise of "don't be concerned about me, I will take care of myself."

After I consoled her into a quieter acceptance of the news, I then made a round of calls to my dearest friends, seeing as I had no family other than Melissa to inform. I spoke to each person in a different manner. Every friend needed an individualized introduction to my new condition. Most reacted with horror. A few friends opined, "God only gives you what you are strong enough to handle." If that were true, I did not like that God. I admit that I did want attention, support, loving concern and validation, and feeling that I was still alive and part of society, but not that I was some chosen scapegoat because I was so "strong." I wanted to feel I was still accepted as an equal by others.

As long as some regarded me as the walking dead, however, I felt excluded from life. This feeling was a *physical* affliction. Had my family of origin been alive during those months, I would not have been able to escape the power of their blanketing victimology over every bit of news I shared. With a bit of guilt, I was thankful they were all dead. I badly needed prayers and empathy from those close to me, not judgment of my "bad luck," which would have smothered me after the diagnosis. But even without my family's mournful predictions for my future, it was easy at this point to be convinced that cancer was just a part of my unlucky path.

At the same time I found myself in denial. Such a strange polarity! I was looking forward to launching a spiritual program so I could mentor a new group of servant leaders in spiritual service. I thought at the beginning of my odyssey I would be able to carry the load of program creator and facilitator plus being a cancer patient. I was falling into part of the cultural dictate that cancer patients often have come to accept: they can continue their lives without interruption. I met many women who did just that, but my experience did not permit such a path. Later in my healing when I began to mentor others with cancer, I heard stories of women who were upset by their families' expectation they should arrange and celebrate extravagant Christmas parties even as they were going through chemotherapy.

In hindsight, I see this polarity of "I am a poor cancer victim" versus "I am just as strong and capable as before" as my tipping point. I had not yet *come to terms* with where I was or what I should be doing, or even feeling. A wonderful term for this is "disorienting dilemma," which connotes going through a major change that will cause me to rethink my life owing to a shift in my values, my identity, and my beliefs. *Illness versus sickness.* There it was. I had an illness called invasive breast cancer, and my culture caused me to see that sickness as making me a cancer victim. But it was now in my hands to determine if that was, indeed, the identity I would adopt.

I had to renegotiate the concept of what a cancer patient might be, and separate the physical illness from the cultural idea of the sickness. I refused to assume personal responsibility for having gotten breast cancer. Yes, I was white, female, older, and had a mother and aunt with mild cases of non-invasive breast cancer. But this didn't point to my personal culpability the way a drinker or smoker might hold himself directly responsible for contracting mouth or lung cancer.

I thought about the psychic damage done to me over the decades by family and superiors, and how those stressors were probably the secondary cause of my cancer. But did that mean I would sit and wallow in self-pity and feelings of helplessness, or was there some other way of constructing a coherent and inclusive perspective of who I was and where I stood in the world at that moment?

Is There a Better Term or Concept?

Once I received my diagnosis, I noted how often other affected people tripped over their tongues trying to share what just occurred. Did they "get" cancer, "have" cancer, were they "stricken" or merely "diagnosed" with cancer? Even more complicated than the verbiage were the various labels. One notable video of cancer patients shows their expression of outrage over the term "cancer victim" (https://www.youtube.com/watch?v=obzooL3Tz8A). Within the cancer community, I read there were new terms floating about such as "cancer thriver," "cancer fighter," "cancer warrior," and "cancer survivor" (although this is a problematic term since there is the possibility of recurrence). None of these terms has yet caught on.

Susan Gubar, in the September 6, 2012, edition of the *New York Times*, also took issue with the phrase as well as the alternatives. "Cancer survivor" is used to connote optimism, yet I felt I would become a survivor of cancer only after having died of a different disease or cause. Gubar adds to this downside by noting that half of those who contract cancer do die from it, so at what point should I feel confident to assert I had survived and am definitely on the other side? I did not feel permanently optimistic, and I decided to refuse to use the term.

I wanted to take a different perspective on what constituted illness, disease, and sickness. Today my husband is fond of saying I "kicked cancers' asses," and at this moment in time, he is right. I am "cancer-free" as of this writing, I am told. But I know that one traitorous cell with the bearing of a suicide bomber might be settling in some organ or bone only to emerge with fury. Not for nothing did the U.S. government label Al Qaida operatives "sleeper cells."

Chambers' English Dictionary defines "patient" as coming from the Latin *pati*, "to bear." It also means a doctor's client. I am still my oncologist's client, and I have borne cancer. So for the time being, until the cultural tides turn and we create a new term for my path, I could say "I have been a cancer patient." It also says to me that I will be *patient* about the course of the disease, and in hoping it never returns, I shall remain both vigilant and courageous.

I'd feel more empowered not to put cancer at the head of any compound term. We "come down with" the flu, colds, a headache, but not cancer. These illnesses are trivial in comparison: they usually do not have high fatality rates, and they are not held in a high psychic or cultural state of fear to the point that the term is whispered.

Bacteria and viruses are also foreign bodies that enter our healthy systems only to have our immune responses overwhelmed. The term "infected with tuberculosis" reflects this alien invasion that does not seem comparable to cancer, where one's cell(s) mutate and attempt to overwhelm the body.

A headache is an internal manifestation, but even the deep pain of a migraine is no match for most cancers. To say I was afflicted with cancer might be closer to the physical and psychological mark. The origin of the word "afflict" comes from the word for "distress," which cancer induces psychologically. But I was looking for a term embracing the totality of the attack on my body: the turning of a normal cell into a rogue killer, the pain and distress of treatment, the discomfort others might feel when speaking to me, and the medical protocols for treatment.

In one sense, I felt the cancer cells, which were my own until they mutated within my body, had committed treason against me. In another sense, I felt as though my mutated cells treated me as a scapegoat. Their desire to live forever, to take over my entire body and kill their host, seemed as egregious a wrong as anything done to me in the serious life situations in which I had been cast.

So was I back to being a cancer *victim*? At this initial phase of my illness, indeed I felt like one. Then I met Barbara Ortiz of the local American Cancer Society. The organization freely uses the phrase "cancer survivor," she explained, because every moment we are alive and functioning as human sentient beings, we have survived what is inside of us or what was removed from within us. I felt relieved to hear this explanation, and am now more comfortable calling myself a cancer survivor today, tomorrow, and beyond.

A Cancer Personality?

Ever since the emergence of the Type A personality discussion, there has been cultural finger-pointing about who develops cancer. Typology discussions have come from a recent finding that might well support certain characteristics as more typical of a cancer patient than others.

Alexander Mostovoy of the Budwig Center holds that there is a carcinogenic personality profile. The people who are the most susceptible to this disease, reports Mostovoy, are those who feel they are bombarded with information regarding cancer. For these people, he says, it is not a question of whether or not they'll get cancer. It is just a matter of when.

The fact that cancer is a multifactorial disease appears to destroy any belief there is one factor alone that might begin its course. First, there is an interplay of activities that lead to the creation of a mutated cell. Second, cancer is usually a slowly progressing disease. Finally, factors such as diet, heredity, environment, lifestyle, personality, and attitude influence when and how a cell might mutate and replicate. With all of these caveats stated, Mostovoy still holds that there is a "carcinogenic personality profile." In general terms, his carcinogenic personality profile can be summed up as follows: loss/grief over a relationship, status, etc.; unfulfilled passion that had been suppressed over many years; unworthiness as a kind soul or "other-centered" someone who puts others' needs before their own; avoidance of conflict by very tidy people; and tension in a parental relationship (Thermography Clinic, Inc.).

This typological profile fails to deal with genetics and multifactorial origins of cancer. The checklist also assures those who do not find themselves on it that they won't get cancer. This is an unwise presentation. It might be true, but it is partial. Conversely, the list is also generic and highly inclusive, which might cause some people to panic. Who cannot point to tension in a parental relationship at some point?

Did my personal history predispose me to cancer? Was I to blame for this misfortune? I believe there are many factors leading to "my" cancer. I had psychological and some environmental factors that might have initiated or accelerated my cancer. Considering this, I no longer felt stuck in the causation dilemma. I could move further into coping with the effects of the *lightning strikes* themselves.

Lightning Strikes

I next looked more closely at my chosen metaphor of *lightning strikes* and clarified it by naming who was being struck and by what. This was a way of making the subject of my initial horror of a diagnosis into an object of consideration, and helped me *come to terms* with what was happening to me. Working with the reality of electrical discharges during a thunderstorm, I adapted the nature of metaphorical lightning strikes as follows:

• A *direct strike*, such as the significant and perhaps fatal injuries sustained by a person from the immediate impact of receiving the diagnosis
• A *contact injury* when a loved one, client, or friend is struck by illness in some manner, and the associate is affected by contact with the loved one's pain
• A *side splash* whereby the loved one, friend, or client has been struck with illness and has taken their pain out on an associate, held him responsible, or projected their pain onto him.

My *lightning strikes* continued to hit me directly over an 18-month period. My family and friends suffered contact injuries, and one friend left after not being able to bear the pain from her closeness to me. I did not cause side splashes directly, but I admit I chose to hold others responsible for the multiple illnesses I endured.

I realized I first had to digest the shock of diagnosis and then collect enough psychic energy to be able to deal with the challenges of the next stage of the healing cycle: *coming to terms*. But this process kept being upended by new strikes, so that phase was delayed time and again. I could not skip navigating the four phases in sequence although I attempted to do so.

My situation was made more complicated by the demands of my teaching obligations and the desire to fulfill my vision of launching a new spiritual program. I now understand that when anyone has experienced a serious life event, it would be wise for the recipient to delay commencing any new and difficult endeavor until the effects of the strike fully manifest. I was so excited by the prospect of bringing my vision to fruition and be of service to others that I rushed the digestion of my diagnosis and failed to appreciate a cancer diagnosis as a major life event. Neglect of self-care would prove to be disastrous to the program.

Once I received the diagnosis, I had to make some crucial decisions: where would I be treated, by whom, and what procedures would I choose to undergo? This pushed me too rapidly into the *coming to terms* stage. The need for haste is a truth of illness, sickness, and the U.S. healthcare system. Of course, there are times where haste is a factor of survival, but even dire situations can be handled with greater sensitivity. My decisions were helped along by my husband's first call after receiving mine. He phoned his close friend, Rich Heller, and then got back to me once I got home that first night.

"Hon? I spoke to Rich," he murmured, in his second call to me, although I believe his soft tone was due more to shock than a desire to shield the contents of the call. "He told me the only place to be treated for breast cancer here in the New York area is at Sloan-Kettering Cancer Center, and we should use the surgeon who operated on his wife."

Upon hearing the name of that renowned cancer hospital, my stomach constricted with fear. I did not truly think my condition was a minor one, but speaking of Sloan-Kettering made me feel as though I were considering hospice care already. *This is the charnel house, the unspeakable name, the place you go when you have been stricken with cancer and are going to die.*

"But I'm being treated at Heights. Dr. Woodward said all I probably need is a lumpectomy and maybe one other treatment. Doesn't sound so serious, so why change doctors and go to Sloan-Kettering?"

Sitting in my kitchen with cell phone in hand, I felt I was occupying two places at once, a spacey feeling of dislocation. *This isn't my place*, I silently affirmed as my body leaned away from my chair. *Not me, not here, I am not meant to have this health problem.*

Even though I resisted the phrase "cancer victim," I couldn't escape the new compound identity of "Lynne with cancer." Having this fearsome disease meant I had to go to a special hospital different from a "normal" hospital because of the severity of my illness. I felt shame in even thinking I had to enter Heights because of cancer. I felt as if everyone who saw me leave the Center knew something toxic and malignant existed within me and would have to be cut out. I felt as though I wore a capital "C" on my jacket.

Now that I was forced to confront the real horror of the diagnosis, where would I best be treated? I felt rushed to find a treatment home. The *lightning strike* had short-circuited my decision-making processes and left them firing along a single track: fear.

Regardless of the severity of the cancer, there must be a way for healthcare practitioners to provide a safe holding environment for the recently diagnosed so they can progress through the *lightning strike* phase quickly and fully. For example, I should not have been left alone to walk out of the cancer center that evening without having been embraced in a more nourishing and receptive environment. I wish I had been provided with pamphlets of hospitals, treatment centers, nutritional information, and healing modalities to help plan my next steps. I needed a patient treatment coordinator or navigator—call it what you will—rather than being left alone with my fears and confusion. What's worse, I went straight from Dr. Woodward's office to my car and into rush hour traffic, which was hazardous to others and me.

I continued to feel dizzy and disoriented even in the safety of my kitchen. What was I to do first? I knew I had little time and energy to develop a plan of action along with Rick. I realize in hindsight my decision came not from any cognitive process, but rather from an emotional center. I had been swayed by the anecdotal success of Rich's wife's treatment, although I did not know what type of cancer she had. Sloan-Kettering was the premier cancer facility in the New York area, and its doctors were rated at the top of their specialties. The hospital offered complementary and alternative medicine (known by the acronym CAM). Complementary medicine involves healing practices *in addition to* the medical standard of care for my cancer. CAM modalities can include acupuncture, yoga, and hypnosis. Alternative medicine treatments, which include practices such as coffee enemas or laetrile, have not been proven in scientifically reliable studies nor are they taught in traditional medical schools.

With this almost magical and superstitious consideration for Sloan-Kettering's status in mind, I decided to switch treatment centers. The next morning I bid the Heights Cancer Center goodbye and made an emergency appointment with Dr. Virgilio Sacchini at Sloan-Kettering; he agreed to become my surgeon.

In my pre-diagnosis life, whenever I found out someone had cancer, I regarded them with the fear that might have been shown by inhabitants of the pre-modern world when spying on lepers, or by the uninformed in the 1980s when they encountered an AIDS patient. I was not alone in this response. Many of my friends reacted to the news of an acquaintance having been diagnosed with cancer with a bowed and shaking head followed by the muttered "poor bastard." What would they be saying about me?

To clear my mind and access a trans-rational perspective, I went to my den where I normally meditate. How would I deal with the *lightning strike* diagnosis and how would I empty my mind to give birth to the next cycle of *coming to terms* with having invasive breast cancer? As with most Western medical practices, I wasn't given much time by my doctor to figure out how I wanted to be treated. Decisions had to be made quickly, and only with a settled mind could I achieve that clarity. I had my personal form of concentrating on my breath. I fell into a quiet state where I might consider a sacred understanding of my life's purpose and destiny. I wanted to access a sense of myself beyond my diagnosis.

During that contemplative time, I saw I was far more than a mastectomy or the statistics I was compiling. I was an ancient part of all that was and is. Some claim that "abracadabra" is among the first words of Genesis, written in Aramaic, and translated as "I will create as I speak." Wilber remarked that Integral Theory provided a way to draw together and thus create an already existing number of ways of seeing reality from different perspectives. By relying on the theory I saw I might create an interrelated network of approaches to my treatment and healing that would be mutually enriching.

In simpler language, by using Integral Theory I could separate out the pre-rational notions that would get in the way of navigating the best course for me to follow, while balancing rational and trans-rational understandings of where I should go and what my life's destiny might entail.

The word *integral* implies the transformation of the entire being, rather than, as in other teachings, just adding more information to the head, or emotional openings for the heart, or practices for the body. Integral Theory seeks a comprehensive understanding of humans and the universe by combining scientific (rational) and spiritual (trans-rational) insights. With my crazy upbringing and damaged sense of self, a lack of community, and a thicket of scientific language to wade through, I would need to aim for total transformation of my entire being.

I reviewed all of my notes on the theory and application as authored by Wilber in over 25 books. Which part was I to address first during these initial frightening hours after my diagnosis? First, I needed to cover what Wilber identified as the master operating system of his framework: quadrants, levels, lines, states, types, and shadow for the model to have a "psychoactive" effect. But integral is not just a to-do list of activities. Using the Integral framework to its full effect depends upon the right intention to be brought to bear, and this intention does not come from the force of ego—and my ego was pretty strongly invested in how forceful it really was.

Instead, I had to connect myself to what I am comfortable calling the Ground of Being. Others might call it the Divine, Spirit, or God. This field is all that is, all that was, and all that will be, and by meditating on it I could deliberately enter into a profound interaction with this Essence.

As I meditated on my breath and my heart, I realized that I wanted to avoid jumping into any one traditional or alternative medical approach without testing it against what I knew of my lived reality. Rather, I wanted to take each medical question and each way of inquiring into that question to see how effective and how pragmatic it would be for my particular cancer and my unique self.

On the other hand, I did not intend to embrace a smorgasbord of unrelated healing modalities. I planned on beginning with the broadest awareness of my situation I could manage while handling my shock. I knew I would also need psychological and spiritual assistance, which I had been unsuccessful in obtaining. I needed the deep psychological assistance which had been offered by my present therapist/guide, Lorraine Antine, who embraced and healed my past psychic traumas. I also needed someone to honor my spiritual position so I could believe that my life was worth fighting for, which was a decision that I had not yet come to fully embrace.

I began with the most basic understanding that humans have toward our situation in the world. There is me, there is you and we, and there is "it" in our body like a bone, or separate from us like a political system or hospital with all of its departments and routines. They are, at base, pronouns: I, We, and It(s). These pronouns are responsible for shaping the three perspectives by which I could begin to understand my newly diagnosed illness.

I first thought about the *first-person, subjective, interior experience* of my feelings and emotions about what was happening to my breast. They are considered first-person because only I can feel them or be aware of them. It is a subjective feeling since they cannot be assessed by a scientific machine. What were my beliefs, hopes, and fears surrounding the fate of this important body part for a woman? Was I so attached to my breast that I would argue for a lumpectomy, or would I want all the possible cancerous tissue removed in a radical mastectomy? How would I feel as a woman, and how would my husband react to this mutilation of my body?

Then I thought about my *second-person, shared experience*, and how my culture, friends, and family would meet with my understanding of my cancer's origins and how to deal with a cure. I would either join in with this shared understanding, or I would have to find another community with which I resonated better. Two friends were horrified that I might opt for surgery, and urged me to go with alternative measures such as herbs and massages. Would I no longer be their friends if I decided to forego alternative treatments for conventional Western medicine? I also had to deal with the culture that surrounded me and within which I existed. Was I unconsciously entrained with its understanding of what causes breast cancer and what might cure it?

Finally, I had to assess and learn more about a *third-person, objective, external, experience* of the realities and human systems that put forth different perspectives. When we talk about the hospital or the procedure of a mastectomy, we are speaking if an "It" or "Its." Imagine the hospital or cancer center that always administers chemotherapy to every patient versus the medical centers that have different criteria for which women undergo the treatment and which do not. Each believes it has "the truth" and is applying only facts, but in reality both are relying on perspectives. So all of these pronouns reflect perspectives rather than absolute truths from any angle we can examine them.

Hospitals can be either parochial or secular; they can carry one particular story of what illness is and how it should be handled, or how they might be guided by experimental efforts. Some hospitals refuse to use blood transfusions due to their religious beliefs, whereas others refuse to end the pregnancy of a patient even if her health would be improved by such a procedure. These are objective, observable systems and structures.

With these three perspectives, I had the start of an approach to healing. But the framework of my task was not the work itself. I would now have to dig deeply into the history of my life and examine who I was at the deepest level. It proved to be a daunting and often depressing task.

CHAPTER TWO

Stress, My Family, and the Early Years

I was born in New York City on July 12, 1945, under the astrological sign of Cancer. My mother Leah was a classic 1940s-style, brown-eyed, brunette beauty with a genius I.Q. and boundless creativity, but she was also besieged by numerous mental illnesses. Leah had married returned-soldier Nathan Rocker two years before my birth. Prior to their wedding, mom had lived with her own mother Anna and her two sisters, Ree and Debbie, in a one-bedroom apartment in Rego Park, Queens. A fourth sister, Elizabeth, had moved out years before to marry Charles and start her family in Philadelphia.

Dad had returned from World War II early in 1943 with an injury to his hearing and bad ulcers. After a torrid romance conducted through censored mail from the Pacific theater of war, dad immediately proposed to mom. They married in the tiny apartment where she had been living with her sisters and mother, and then settled into a two-bedroom apartment in nearby Forest Hills, New York.

Once Leah became pregnant with me in 1944, her high blood pressure threatened both of our lives. She spent June of 1945 in the hospital due to pre-eclampsia, a severe condition that was potentially life threatening for both of us. Mom's high blood pressure rendered her susceptible to a stroke, and caused problems with the functioning of my placenta. We were both under significant physical stress that last month, which my mother claimed was exacerbated by second-rate medical care.

"I had such a dumb doctor! All of the good ones were still overseas treating the soldiers, so we ladies got the dregs. The idiot x-rayed me and said there was a shadow behind you, and I was supposed to be having twins. It was so disappointing when only one of you showed up. I kept asking him what happened to the other one."

Twin fantasies plagued me thereafter: where was that sibling who could help me navigate the crazy world I'd been born into?

"They had to *cut* me," my mother would continue her story to visitors, with me quietly listening at her knee, and proceed to exclaim with great drama, "Then I *bled!*"

Of course, I felt horribly guilty as a little child hearing my birth was responsible for my mother's month-long hospitalization, her possible stroke and/or death, and then finally for her mutilation and bleeding—all just to usher me into the world. She never corrected my misapprehension that I was responsible for this painful situation.

For years I thought I had been a Caesarian birth, but when I had my own child, I realized mom had referenced her episiotomy, a routine, small incision that permits the baby to come out without tearing vaginal tissue. I was a breech baby, exiting feet and bum first, so an episiotomy made sense. Later I found out my mother had been anesthetized throughout the entire delivery anyhow.

My mom was the second of six children born to Grandma Anna Neuman and her husband, Lazarus David Greenberg. Tall, handsome, and brilliant, Lazarus was expected to become a rabbi. He moved from his family home in Romania to Germany in order to study at an Orthodox yeshiva, but while in Germany, Lazarus learned of a new branch of the Jewish religion called Reform. Preferring this more liberal interpretation of his faith, my grandfather moved first to Philadelphia—where he met and married my grandmother— and then to Cincinnati, where he hoped to attend Hebrew Union College to become an ordained Reform rabbi. However, Lazarus soon announced he no longer believed in God, and thereafter made a meager living as a jeweler in a tiny shop across the street from the seminary while debating Torah with the students.

My mother told me Lazarus suffered several nervous breakdowns during his life before fleeing south to form another family. He didn't bother divorcing his shy little wife Anna or caring for their six children. Inhibited Ree was the eldest. My mother, the beautiful tomboy, came next. Then came two boys, Sol and Danny, who were unknown to me until I was seven. Aunt Elizabeth had been a great beauty in her youth, married Charles, and had two children, Steven and Leslie, my cousins, whom I never knew. Then there was the baby of the crew, Aunt Debbie, who was 16 years older than me, short and stout as a dumpling with an explosive temper. I was told that Lazarus, for whom I was named, eventually died of lung cancer after a lifetime of smoking unfiltered cigarettes.

***

When we moved from Queens in 1950 to Long Island, my mother expanded information about her family whenever she was in her storytelling mood. I knew there was something mysterious about my two missing uncles, because whenever my two aunts mentioned "Danny" or "Sol," they hushed one another. One day I asked mom who Danny and Sol were, and why they weren't around to be part of our tiny family.

"They were my younger brothers, Lovey, and oh how gorgeous and brilliant they both were! But one day Danny was playing with Sol with a spoon, pretending the spoon was a bayonet. He lunged at Sol—they were just little boys, in their early teens—and Danny accidentally gouged out Sol's eye. When my father got home he was so outraged at the mutilation of his gorgeous blond-haired, blue-eyed son that he raged at my brother Danny until Dan ran out of the house, never to return. We later learned that Danny settled nearby, but he never spoke with anyone in the family again."

Mom stared at her folded hands and I saw tears appear in her soft brown eyes. Tears were not a rarity for my mother, but something about that moment melted my heart and I empathetically reached out to comfort her.

"Sol was so heartbroken over his brother's exile that he left home soon after. No one ever knew if he survived or what actually happened to him."

"Don't cry, Mommy." I was a devastated daughter of five then, and I hugged her tightly. "We'll find Uncle Sol someday."

From then on, wherever we traveled we looked up every Solomon Greenberg in the phone book and called them to see if they were mom's long-lost brother. I fantasized that I would get grandma on the TV show "Queen For A Day," and when they put the crown on her head, Sol would rush out and they would tearfully embrace.

⊙⚜ ⚜☉

Shortly after my sixth birthday, I was kneeling on the couch in an airless apartment in Queens combing my grandmother's luxurious long grey hair. I went into an altered state as I brushed and braided it. While grandma stayed still and silent during my ministrations, my mother and her two sisters were puttering in the high-ceilinged kitchen around the old-fashioned claw-foot sink, but soon began bickering in tones that could have passed for angry songs. I was only paying half-attention to what was being said until I heard raised voices.

"How *dare* you go off and marry *him*?" Aunt Debbie shouted. That "him" referred to my father who was sitting on a chair by the TV reading the sports section.

Neither my mother nor my aunts seemed to care if he heard the insult or not, but my head jerked over to assess my daddy's reaction to this insult. My father, whose hearing had been damaged in the war, simply turned down the volume of his hearing aid, and continued reading the paper. I was now alert to the growing discord in the kitchen.

"I had to get out of here with you and Ree always dragging me down," my mother snorted. "I make sure Nat gives me money so I can give it to you. What an ungrateful person you are! Otherwise I'd be stuck here with all of you making *no* money."

Debbie flung off the beautifully detailed apron Grandma had sewn for her on the old pedal-style sewing machine, and stormed into the living room. She swung around to face my mother who was at the kitchen sink and retorted in a shrill tone, "I'm *suffering* because of *you*! You dragged us away from Cincinnati where we had relatives, people who could help us, not this godforsaken Queens with kikes all around me. I'm not living any type of life, and where

42

are the babies suckling from these breasts?" She held up her ample breasts for emphasis.

"Don't you *dare* pull that on me." My mother's nostrils flared, like an animal prior to charging. "I gave up marrying two multi-millionaires in order to continue working and keep a roof over your head. I slaved along with Ree painting greeting cards right here in this one bedroom horror until my hands ached and my sight blurred!"

"You're such a fool, Leah," Debbie countered in a low, menacing tone. "You should have married one of those rich men and then mom and I would be taken care of the way we should have been." Debbie ran shaking into the one bedroom and slammed the door shut with such force the apartment shuddered.

Aunt Ree, two years older than my mother, was porcelain-skinned and dainty. She reminded me of the pen illustrations in my grandmother's Civil War books. I could imagine her in vast swaths of crinolines fluttering a fan. But even this shy and retiring lady joined in the cacophony of complaints.

"How *could* you do that to poor Debbie? You know how hard she works keeping the apartment clean for mom and me. She's a *slave* here and you had to leave us to marry Nat! How selfish could you be, Leah?"

When my mother started to cry, I stopped brushing my grandmother's hair. Debbie was sobbing in the bedroom; my grandmother couldn't hear much of what had transpired because her hearing was impaired, so she just looked confused; and my dad heaved sighs of silent frustration. It was time for this vulnerable only and lonely child to go home.

⚜

My mother had painted the walls of my tiny bedroom to look like a forest filled with mythical creatures. I was surrounded by unicorns that hid behind lush forests and fairies that peeked through tree branches. When she tucked me in at night she would repeat the story of her family; she always instructed me that my own chapter was yet to be written.

"Long, long ago in Austria," she began in fairy-tale fashion, "lived your great-grandmother, and she worked for the Empress."

Such promising magical beginnings excited me into visions of ball gowns and tiaras. Her melodic singsong continued:

"Your great-grandmother fell in love with your great-grandfather, but her family was against their marriage. So she went to the Empress and asked for her help. The Empress was so impressed by their love that she gave them a pair of diamond and gold earrings. The couple decided to run away to America where they could marry, and use these priceless earrings for their new life together."

By now I was in full thrall and to this day I can conjure up a mental image of those wondrous earrings.

"Where are the earrings now, Mommy?" I prodded.

"Your great-grandmother gave those gorgeous earrings to her first-born child, your very own grandma Anna."

"But where are they *now*?"

"Your great-grandmother died when grandma was eight and her younger brother Joseph was only six."

I could never get comfortable in my bed at this point. I'd kick at the bed sheets and look at a unicorn to try to comfort myself.

"Your great-grandfather wanted a new wife to care for him and he quickly remarried a widow with her own children. The new woman didn't want to care for grandma and her brother, but she *did* want those earrings. So she kept the earrings and threw grandma and Uncle Joe out of the house and into the street. They were on their own and had nothing. It was winter and the wind was howling and your grandma was in charge of her little brother but with nowhere to go."

After that dramatic ending, my mother kissed me goodnight. I was left with visions of real-life wicked stepmothers and homeless children alone in the freezing cold. As I got older I came to understand that mom's family, me included, was subjected to some type of curse named after her maiden name. "The Curse of the Greenbergs," my mother called it. Although I never believed in actual curses, I did have a nascent understanding of karma, and therefore the idea of perpetual bad luck made a certain kind of sense to me.

Dad and mom's marriage was certainly not stable; it had quiet valleys and then stormy peaks where the subject of divorce flew out of mom's mouth in a stream. Whenever my mother went into a tirade about divorcing dad, I always went into a panic. My earliest memory of these explosions happened while driving on Long Island, while we were taking one of our pleasure rides to the shore. It was a rainy yet mild fall day, and our plan was to look at the ocean. Classical music streamed through static on the car radio. The thrum of raindrops on the window lulled me into a pleasant reverie in the back seat until my mother's shrill voice interrupted the music.

"I hate you!" she burst out. "You're a complete disappointment to me!"

I realized this was aimed at my father and would only escalate. There was nowhere to hide. So I tightly grasped my dolly, Gretel, and stroked her curly reddish-blonde hair.

"Ahhh, here we go again," my father muttered. I could see his hands tighten on the steering wheel.

"Don't you *dare* talk to me that way. You know you could have finished college at NYU on the G.I. bill, but you were too *stupid* to take advantage of it, like your family."

That last phrase puzzled me even at my young age. I knew my father's family had gone to a college called Cornell. I kissed Gretel's porcelain face and looked out the window at the drops scurrying down the glass.

"So who am I married to?" From the passenger's seat in the front Mom pounded the dashboard with her fist. "A *shmata* [dry goods] salesman who doesn't make any money—that's all you are! I deserve better. Look who I gave up! Two brilliant multi-millionaires, only to wind up with *you*."

I kept my eyes on Gretel's porcelain face and stared into her unblinking eyes as if to find solace there.

"I'll take Lynne Donna and move back in with my sisters. You can do whatever you want."

Suddenly the back seat of the black Ford seemed to have shrunk. The car felt cold, despite the pleasant rainy autumn day. Shivering,

I thought sadly of having to leave my apartment, my room with the unicorns mommy had painted all over my walls, and my canary. I didn't want to live in that crowded one bedroom with my constantly bickering aunts. I didn't want to leave my daddy.

I seemed to separate from the back seat of the Ford and float up through my body, right out the top of my head. Emerging at the Long Island shore in an ethereal apparition, I felt the warmth of the summer sun fall on my face; the sand was fine and granular beneath the soles of my bare feet and between my toes. Instead of my parents' arguing, I heard the music of the waves lapping at the shore. I had thus begun to "relocate," which I had perfected as a defense mechanism by the time I found myself in Dr. Woodward's office.

⚓ ⚓

When I was 10 years old my mother's mental health began to deteriorate. Mom had a total hysterectomy but received no hormone replacement therapy. The sudden and complete lack of estrogen triggered a nervous breakdown, and mom was treated with an early version of electroshock therapy. When she returned from these treatments, I hid in the basement. The woman who returned from the hospital that night was not my mother, I was sure. When my dad dragged mom up the stairs to their second floor bedroom, her voice sounded dead as she whimpered nonsensical phrases. I dared to peek up from the top step of the basement. I pressed my face against the cold cinder blocks and eyed my mother who displayed a frightening bloated face; so different from the mother I knew who had left for the hospital in the morning.

Leah's mental health vacillated over the years. She became fragile again when I was eleven and the three of us moved to Dallas in 1956. Dad had been promoted to southwest regional vice-president of his textile firm. In addition to a raise, we were entitled to rent new Cadillacs every two years and join the Jewish country club at company expense. But it also meant dad would have to travel five days a week for months at a time to oversee his company's accounts. Mom felt stranded from the cultural dislocation of having to fit into a Southwestern town. For the first time in 20 years, she no longer had the security of her sisters and mother to push back against. None of our neighbors or erstwhile new friends would put up with her mood shifts and odd behavior, so she remained isolated with only me for company.

Almost immediately after our move, my mother became fixated on Grace Kelly, the American actress, who was preparing to wed Prince Rainier of Monaco. Mom obsessed and raged over Kelly for months while the news and ladies' magazines featured numerous stories about this American film star who was becoming a true royal princess.

"It's not *fair!*" my mother railed. "Look at *her*! Look at *me*! Aren't I more beautiful than Grace Kelly?" she demanded of me as we watched news of the upcoming nuptials on TV. "*I* should have been married to someone rich and important. *I* deserve to be treated like a queen. Why am I mopping floors and darning your father's socks?" she demanded, looking from me to my father. "Where's the prince who's supposed to take *me* away?"

She took off her wedding ring and flung it on the bedroom floor where it landed at my father's feet. Dad and I stood frozen at the outburst, but he finally picked up the delicate ring I had long admired.

"That ring…" she sputtered, "That ring is *nothing*." It had one center stone of a half carat and two smaller ones on either side set in platinum. "Other women were given huge rocks by their husbands. Where's mine?" She faced my father in a boiling rage as the slight droning of an airplane's engine was heard flying somewhere nearby. It must have been a reasonable distance from our home, but the engine was still audible. "What about *that*?" she folded her new complaint seamlessly into her litany. Pointing in the direction of the noise, she pummeled us with every word. "Will you listen to that damn plane? Who can live with a roar like that constantly overhead without getting ill?"

Dallas Love Field, our commercial airport, was located 30 minutes away. A recent change in landing patterns had caused occasional incoming flights to fly close enough for a faint rumbling to be heard.

"I sent Love Field a letter telling them they're driving me crazy with their new flight pattern," mom announced, storming into our kitchen. She opened a cupboard, removed some cans and shut the cabinet door with a bang. "Next I'm going to write letters to the Dallas *Morning News* about how I'm suffering." Crash went a skillet onto the range. "I'm going to have another breakdown!" Grace Kelly and the wedding ring were now temporarily forgotten.

"Mom, they don't care about you or that you're upset," I tried. "Wear earmuffs or something. The noise isn't even loud enough to rattle the plates." I collected the silverware to set the table.

"I'm a sensitive artist," my mother replied, "and my nerves are very easily upset. I can't sleep at night just thinking about the awful noises I'm going to hear tomorrow. *They* have to change where they land those goddamn planes!"

Perhaps spring boarding from the "Battle of Love Field," my mother's next obsession was the eradication of all mention of plane crashes. Scared of flying, she demanded my father and I cut out every plane crash story from the newspapers so her day would not be disturbed by alarming information. We complied without question. After that, newspapers often resembled a patchwork string of grey paper dolls.

"Won't she realize that every cut out space means another plane crash?" I asked my father as we sat at the kitchen table snipping away.

"You know your mother," he said without looking up. "Just keep cutting."

⚬⚮⚬

The following year, 1957, when I turned 12, mom slipped into a severe depression and slept continuously while curled up in a fetal position on her bed. For the next two years, I tip-toed around my depressed mother, and tried to pretend that everything was all right at school. I was beginning to learn that I had an odd family and felt it my duty to prevent others from finding out just how odd it was. None of my friends were privy to my mom's condition; I became resourceful in making up creative excuses as to why she wasn't up and about cleaning or chauffeuring me to events. I came up with enough excuses to get rides from friends' parents when I needed to go somewhere. In fact, pretending became my favorite activity.

In those years I took up acting and found I had an uncanny gift of pretending to be someone else and to be somewhere else.

But no amount of pretending could conceal my mother's condition on one particular afternoon in 1959. It was shortly after my fourteenth birthday when my mother's status was abruptly telegraphed to our tight neighborhood. Leah suddenly announced she wanted to die, ran naked out of her bathroom, and headed for the front door of our house. Out the door, across the manicured lawn with the banks of gardenia bushes in full bloom, and down the sidewalk she bolted toward a busy intersection as fast as a colt. No words needed to be spoken between my dad and me. He paused only to retrieve mom's coat before racing out the door after her. I stopped at the threshold, my gaze transfixed on the naked figure of my mother running through the main street of our neighborhood.

I couldn't feel anything; I went numb, watching my athletic dad sprint after my mother. I felt nothing when he caught up to her and threw the coat over her shoulders. I didn't hear the words he spoke softly while leading her back to the safety of our house. Tenderly, Dad put her to bed. We nodded woodenly to one another, and I retired into my room. Later, I paced around my bed and wondered what had happened to my mother. What had made her bolt out of the house naked and race down our residential street? She had seemed withdrawn but not angry before the event occurred. Why would she want to die? After that incident, mom's psychiatrist urged her to spend a month in a psychiatric facility and receive more shock treatments. She left that day for in-patient care.

My classmates had only one other "deviant" family to fathom in our upper middle class neighborhood of brick ranch homes, and that was a divorced couple—marital splits were unheard of in our community in those days. My situation made me an outstanding target for mockery; even the hiring of a nanny to care for me during my mother's month-long hospitalization provided great fodder for my classmates' nasty repartee.

"Where's your mother?" a classmate, Ellen Shapiro, taunted me in junior high.

Unschooled in the ways of the retort or simple lying, I lamely countered, "She's in theBeverly Hills Rest Home and Sanitarium, but she's in the *rest home* part."

Ellen already knew where my mother was, but—like the other kids in school who cornered me with the same question—she delighted in seeing me squirm. "What's she need a *rest* from?" Ellen laughed. "You?"

Back home six weeks later, my mother attempted to settle into a normal routine.

"I'm sorry, Lynne Donna," she said upon her return, "I know I'm your mother, but I can't remember your birthday."

I helped her remember, but the gaps about how to parent me and who I was remained.

Looking back today with twenty-twenty hindsight, I see that I was always trying to please my mother—an impossible achievement. Lacking effective maternal recognition from her, I found substitute satisfaction by becoming active in many different school and extracurricular groups. I filled my days and nights with organizational activities, participating in the groups' contests in acting and writing, and I began to win numerous honors and awards. If I had to stick out at school, I reasoned, at least let it be for accomplishments. With no siblings or cousins, I relied on friendships, but these tended not to extend beyond the group to which I belonged. Other girls had friendships with the children of their parents' close friends. Entire families would go on vacation or celebrate holidays together so the girls were always surrounded by their peers, but that was not possible for me.

In those days, I lived with the fear that my mother would contract bronchitis, or her most feared enemy, cancer. It never entered my mind that I might be a cancer patient a half century later. Mostly, back then, there was no time to think of myself, as mom and her challenges loomed so large in my life. Adolescence, the great time of doubts and uncertainties for all normal teenagers, was excruciating for me and yet, quite simply, there was no time for me.

I often heard the story about why my mother married my father after not marrying her two multi-millionaire beaus, and I already knew she considered this choice to be the biggest mistake of her life.

"I chose to marry your father not because I loved him, but because he was an athlete. He had this jaunty carriage. I figured my children would inherit my looks and your father's strong constitution. But you look like your father and got my bad health. What a disappointment."

I did indeed look more like my dad than her cinematically proportioned beauty. When I was fifteen she informed me I was getting a nose job so mine would look more like her pert little upturned one. I had not thought at the time that my nose needed reshaping, but off we went to the plastic surgeon.

"Well," the merry doctor welcomed me, "So why do you want plastic surgery on your nose at such a young age?"

Since it was not my idea, I had no answer for him, and I silently looked hard over at my mother for her to fill in the information gap. The doctor saw my blank look and then responded, "I will not take your case, Lynne Donna, since I can tell this isn't your wish at all."

We left. My mother had been thwarted, and I felt badly for having been the source of her sour mood. A week later the pictures of me around the house mysteriously achieved penciled nose jobs where my mother had shaded away the bulk and length to do via art that which she couldn't do in reality.

⚯⚯

My safety in the world as a socially active teen was, like everything else, directed by my mother.

"You can't trust people, Lynne Donna, especially boys," mom reminded me as we sat together at the kitchen table shucking corn the day before my date with fellow 10th grader Jimmy Stark. She stopped ripping off the husks to tap the table for emphasis. "There isn't one single person in this world besides me and your aunts and grandma that you can trust." She was in full authority mode as her eyes bored into my head. "You must call me two times during your date, do you understand? If you don't call, I'll get sick from worry."

"Mom, for God's sake, don't make me hunt up coin phones wherever I am," I protested, knowing it would have no weight with her.

"You wouldn't want to make me sick or die from worry, would you?" Now she laced her fingers on top of the cornhusks and leaned forward for emphasis. "Remember, don't believe anything other people tell you. No one loves you as much as your mother. And besides, you know your mother is always right."

❧ ❧

"Your mother is always right." I had felt enmeshed with and smothered by my mother and her family as I was growing up, but her illnesses, both physical and psychological, left me hovering around her in a genuine caring mode. The natural separation between us would occur when I left for college, I felt sure, since wasn't that a natural time for teens to declare their independence?

Like my other Jewish friends, after graduating in 1963, I only applied to the University of Texas in Austin. I would be among friends I'd socialized with for many years. I was known by Jewish teens from all around Texas, having competed in acting and oratorical contests during high school at one of the numerous synagogue and organizational gatherings. I was well liked by this group of Jewish youth, and dreamed that the bullying and teasing I experienced in high school from the other students could be erased and a fresh start implemented. In those days it was imperative to join a sorority since the campus in Austin had 40,000 students and a freshman class of 10,000. These groups were organized along racial and religious lines. To be excluded from one of these groups in 1963 was to be relegated to outcast status.

Off I went for the weeklong pre-registration event known as "rush." My dad lugged a huge steamer trunk into my tiny dorm room and I got acquainted with Betsy, my new roommate. Betsy and I didn't attempt to learn much about one another since once we were pledged to our respective sororities we were expected to bond exclusively with them. I can't even remember what she looked like.

Things were going well during the sorority rush mixers until the final offer of membership was to appear in our mailbox. To my horror, out of all of the Jewish freshmen, only a girl who had a baby during high school and I were not invited to join any of the three Jewish sororities. I felt as though my life was over. I would forever be lumped at the bottom of the social strata with the one poor girl who had a baby out of wedlock, which was the ultimate shame back then. No frat boy would ever date me as a "GDI," an unintentional God Damn Independent of "questionable" repute. How and why did this happen to me? Were my family and I indeed cursed as my mother always hinted, or was there something intrinsically wrong with me? What made no sense was the fact that despite my mother's interference, I had led a lively high school social life and had been embraced by a cadre of loyal friends with interests similar to my own.

I sat in my dorm room with my head in my hands, not moving for hours after failing to receive a bid to join a Jewish sorority. I examined the ruin of my young life as all of the other girls left for their pledging ceremonies. I couldn't foresee a future for myself now. Would I wander alone amidst the huge campus without a friend? I had no religious or coherent philosophical belief system to either be shattered or give me succor. I had no thoughts of suicide, but I felt distant from myself, numb and confused. I blamed myself for being rejected by the social heart of my college. There had to be something wrong with me.

At dinner later that night as the girls returned from their ceremonies, all my old friends wore their pledge pins, and they sat with their new sorority "sisters." I did indeed wander alone through the huge dining hall. But I refused to let them see me cry. I put on a cheery, buoyant persona I had created long ago for such soul-crushing moments as this. I sashayed down the rows of chatting sorority cliques with a book in hand, sat down at an empty table, and created the ambiance of a young woman happily engrossed in a captivating novel. I forced my eyes to scan down the left page and then to the top of the right one, never aware of a word within my field of vision. I placed all of my distraught emotions into a jar and sealed it with paraffin wax; never would I permit these honest sorrows to leak out anywhere at any time.

But alone in my room that evening, amidst wrenching sobs, I phoned home and brought the news to my folks. My parents could not understand how their daughter—who had done all the "right" things, belonged to all of the "right" groups, and who had an impressive résumé—would be so ostracized. Mom and Dad went to our Rabbi Klein and asked him to inquire around our local Jewish community to see if he could discern the reason I had been shunned.

When Rabbi Klein reported back the next day, they were stunned. He told them to drive down to Austin and bring me home from college immediately because my life might be in danger from a girl I had known in high school, Mary Anne Roth.

"Mary Anne apparently hates Lynne Donna because of Lynne's singular success at Hillcrest High as an actress," he began. "Seems that Mary Anne wanted those starring roles that your daughter won, but she never was assigned even a small role."

My father shared this information with me as he told me he was driving down to Austin immediately to take me home. I could only dimly recall Mary Anne and her auditions for our high school plays year after year. She would stand off stage biting her nails before each of her dismal auditions, but no one ever took her seriously as an actress.

Later, my parents told me Rabbi Klein had offered more detail in a second phone call. "Did you know she has a violent streak?" he asked my parents. "Mary Anne stabbed her mother in the back with a knife when she was still in high school," the rabbi continued. "I don't know how they covered this up. Once she got to UT, she made up ugly stories about Lynne Donna impugning every aspect of her life. That's how Mary Anne managed to get your daughter blackballed from all three Jewish sororities." He concluded, "I'm really afraid she might continue her hatred of your daughter and put Lynne's life at risk."

My dad drove down to Austin right after he ended the call with Rabbi Klein. We hurriedly repacked my trunk. I did not speak to my roommate of one week to explain my departure or to say goodbye, nor did she ask me why I was leaving. I glanced for the last time at my dorm room mirror and saw a pale face devoid of emotion or hope. I silently vowed that I would get back at Mary Anne by living a productive and successful life, albeit one where I would never permit myself to show sorrowful or hurt emotions.

Alone in the back seat of our Cadillac that night heading home, I realized I was returning to Dallas with no plans for my freshman year. Concerned that I would waste an entire year of my life, the next morning I raced over to Southern Methodist University (SMU), a few miles from my home, and begged them to admit me. After hearing my story, the compassionate administrative dean accepted me on the spot, and I began my college career as a full-time commuter student the following day. I felt as though I had entered the witness protection program; I needed protection from harm from familiar sources, and SMU was a totally unknown arena to me.

It was many years before I could consider the threatening event at UT in a more objective light. As a mature woman I realized I had been targeted by a mentally ill girl; something that could have happened to any student. But at eighteen, my past psychological abuse by my mother rendered me vulnerable to thinking I was just the type of person who others want to victimize. I became hypervigilant toward people after this episode, accustomed as I was to my own mother's constant changes of behavior from loving to psychologically abusive. I came to understand when a friend would unexpectedly turn on me. Over the years, as seldom as it occurred, I realized that being on the wrong side of a vengeful person who possessed no empathy was far more the other person's burden than my own. I have kept this realization with me through today.

When I received my cancer diagnosis in 2010, it was no stretch to interpret the damning news as just another part of my intensely lived life. Like a chain of paper dolls, each negative event appeared as the next figure hanging in sequence and forming a sad tableau.

⁂

I had no intention of remaining at SMU for my entire undergraduate education. I spent a productive year there while preparing to transfer in my sophomore year. My first choice was to transfer to Newcomb College of Tulane University (a woman's coordinate college like Radcliffe was attached to Harvard, or Barnard to Columbia). When I was accepted to Newcomb in 1964, the college was still legally segregated by race and gender. I didn't care. I had fallen in love with constitutional law, and heard of a professor at Newcomb, Alexander Lacy, who was extraordinarily gifted in this area. I wanted him as my professor.

Newcomb was the college to which all female candidates had to apply, and where they took classes the first two years. This permitted Southern girls to stretch their intellectual and leadership wings. In the South in the mid-1960s, the dominant thinking still emphasized that an intellectual girl would frighten off Southern men. It was bad enough that I, a strong, tall, Southern woman, dreamed of becoming a lawyer. But Newcomb was a haven for forward-thinking women who thought they had the right to be leaders and the right to be smart.

New Orleans could not have been more different from Dallas. Dallas was a "dry" county where individual drinks could not be purchased; in New Orleans, booze flowed to anyone tall enough to reach the bar. Dallas was predominantly Southern Baptist, while New Orleans was genteel Old South Roman Catholic. Dallas had a basically arid former cotton-growing ecology, whereas New Orleans was lush with semi-tropical growth. The mostly hot, moist climate fostered unfathomable perfumes that burst forth from riots of floral blossoms. The air seemed edible to me. The French Quarter featured a cornucopia of aromas: gardenias and bougainvillea, *café au lait*, and the irresistible odor of beignets, or deep-fried choux pastry. The wrought-iron fences interspersed with top-ranked restaurants provided lascivious peeks into the elegant and debauched gatherings of New Orleans' haute society. On weekends we students treated ourselves to repasts at famous eateries such as Antoine's, Gallatoire's, The Court of Two Sisters, Brennan's, and Commander's Palace. Without the aid of marijuana, I could be transported into altered states just wandering the streets and absorbing what the air and my senses provided.

In my first real dorm experience, I finally learned how other girls had been raised by their parents, and was forced to absorb the fact that my upbringing did not resemble any norm. For example, my mother had abilities that astonished and confounded me, and she was often asked by professors at SMU to demonstrate her powers while under self-hypnosis. Mom could write different sentences with each hand simultaneously, and not bleed when her arm was pierced with a knitting needle. (When she was 87 she had eye surgery while under hypnosis. She chatted amicably with the surgeons who were cutting her lower eyelids off and experienced neither pain nor bleeding.) Mom would put herself into an altered state in order to discover items she had lost. She recovered a misplaced valuable brooch by putting herself into a trance and then walking straight to the brooch's resting place. My father, a staunch non-believer in mystical states, blanched upon seeing her enter the room with auras dancing around her head and the brooch in her palm. These abilities began at a very young age, and were confirmed by my aunts. She was also a consummate and international award winning author of poetry and short stories; adept at needlepoint, knitting, oil and water color painting, and dressmaking; cooking; and playing the piano without ever having a lesson. The girls adored my stories of my mother's psychic abilities, her adventures under hypnosis, and her incredible creativity.

But the girls were also able to mirror back my mother's unhealthy dominance and how I was tied to her emotional states. A happy Leah resulted in a happy Lynne, and a depressed Leah meant a depressed Lynne. I became confused; was my mother great or evil? Was I damaged goods or a fortunate only child? When a domineering mother is a potent mix of charisma and instability, what happens to the daughter? But instead of seeking expert advice from a therapist, I repressed my questions and reveled in a busy college life in New Orleans. I immediately began to synthesize the effect of culture on its art in my art history class and then do the same with my English class. Was everything related to everything else?

≈≈

Professor Lacy's constitutional law class proved to be just what I had hoped it would be: scintillating and challenging. I was one of the top two students in the class, along with Celine Weinberg, and we quickly bonded as best friends. I was also the top student in a class on Spanish mystic poets. It was there that I found I had inherited something from my mother's unusual portfolio of talents: I intuitively understood mysticism. But unlike other students, I failed to embrace the growing fascination with Eastern mystics, and stuck to Judeo-Christian philosophy. By then I was a cultural Jew who attended High Holy Day services, although I was not active in any other Jewish observances on campus. My mystical exercises came from my own understandings and experiences.

Marijuana hit the Tulane campus in 1964, and of course I joined in experimenting with it. But I found I could create my own highs by simple shifts of conscious awareness, and smoked it less and less until I stopped all together. With natural blond hair and yellow-hazel eyes, I would don a yellow blouse and yellow slacks and "disappear" into a different zone for hours at a time. While in this self-created high I felt joined with all creation with nothing separating me from anything or anyone else. It then took another simple shift of conscious awareness to return to normal functioning. This was a different state of interiority than my ability to dissociate, which enabled me to escape and protect myself during times of severe stress. The ability to "get high" connected me with a bliss-state I had never encountered previously. None of my friends could understand what I was doing without the aid of pills, pot, or other substances. This forced me to keep my adventures to myself. These peeks into another way of perceiving the world excited me immensely. They called me to attempt to join what my education decreed were polarities that could never be reconciled: science and mysticism.

Along with sorority sisters Bebe, Louise, and Angela, we set up a little think tank in the cafeteria and tried to integrate the experiences we were all encountering through various drugs with what our studies were teaching us about the "real world." A month of such heady evenings brought us no closer to completing our proposed project and we decided to suspend our search. These endeavors were a welcome diversion from trying to figure out how to deal with my mother's mental illness and her peculiar way of instructing me on how to live my life.

I had another cousin whom I never knew, even though she lived across the street from my aunts and grandma. She was Aunt Ann's only child, Sharon, my father's only niece. We two never interacted because neither family wanted to mix with the other. My father's family found my mother and aunts to be crazy and isolated, and my mother's family considered their Sephardic Jewish background to be superior to my father's background from Eastern Europe. According to my mother, "The Rockers are beneath us and there's no reason for you to mix with them." With one exception when I was six, the two of us never shared time together or spoke to one another.

When Cousin Sharon announced her engagement, she was twenty-four and I was nineteen. I flew home from Tulane, and then mom, dad, and I flew to New York to celebrate her nuptials. It was perhaps the third time I would have seen my cousin. Since I was not permitted to buy my own clothes until I was almost twenty, mom selected a dress for me from the fashionable Lillie Rubin store. Although it was beautiful, it made me look matronly. My mother, who had a fantastic figure, insisted on buying herself a black dress more appropriate for a funeral than a reception.

"No, no, please Leah," my dad beseeched her. "Wear the lovely peach dress with the flowers that you brought. You look like a model in it."

"God, mom, you'll insult them and no one will speak to us!" I screamed.

But her true motivation for donning it came out right before we left for the wedding.

"Why isn't it *you* getting married instead of her?" she suddenly shrieked at me over her shoulder which caused me to shake.

Attempting a rational argument I responded, "Because I'm only nineteen and I haven't fallen in love yet, mom."

It was a flat answer devoid of emotion. I had long ago repressed anger toward my mother and couldn't make a stronger case about the marriage accusation. To point out its absurdity would have been too dangerous, as I had learned from countless occasions.

She swung around to face me as she was finishing her makeup in the hotel bathroom. "You will *never* get married. You don't know how to attract a man! All the other girls know how! Sharon is from your father's family and even *she* managed to snag a fellow, an elementary school principal at that, so why can't you?"

I had no answer. I looked down at the rug. My father exhaled loudly in exasperation but made no attempt to deflect the irrational tirade or come to my defense.

Her last insult pierced me deeply: "*If you ever manage to get married, it will be to a shoe salesman!*"

With tears streaming down my face, I turned away from her and completed getting ready. My mother had spoken; her curse had been flung.

At the reception that night my father's entire family shunned my mother and us for my mother's obvious "fuck you" symbol of wearing a graveside black dress on their happiest day. None of them ever forgot that insult, and I was pretty much alienated from my dad's side of the family thereafter.

A week later I was back in college and my folks were home in Dallas. Still stinging from my mother's prophecy, I phoned her to ask why she had made that particularly nasty remark. "Why, Lynne Donna, you and your father and I had a *lovely* time at Sharon's wedding. I don't know what you're talking about."

⁓⁓

My father was hopelessly in love with his gorgeous, brilliant, and limitlessly talented wife, and he stayed with mom even as her humiliations and rages rained on his back. He was a confused "normal" husband who just couldn't figure out what was wrong with his beautiful, albeit unstable, wife. He was often away on business during the week and when he returned home, he sought refuge on the golf course on weekends.

"Honey," he phoned me one weekend in 1965 when I was twenty and in the midst of the spring semester at Tulane, "How about coming home next weekend? Don't worry about the plane tickets, I'll cover them. You need to do what only you can do, and you do so

60

well. Your mom's depressed and you know how happy she gets when you come home."

"Daddy, it's the Sigma Alpha Mu formal next weekend. I've got a date, a dress, and a hair appointment."

"Then free up the next weekend, okay? You're the only one who can make her happy, you know that. Do your old dad a favor and make sure you come home then."

Such was my role in the world: to make it a happier place for my mother, and to give her my successes, which flowed in consistently, to shore up her ego.

"After all," she had reminded me repeatedly, "I had you for *me*, not for anyone else. Your father didn't care about having you, it was *me*."

The catch was I could never adequately fulfill that special role.

⚘

I chose to attend Columbia University's Graduate Faculties in Public Law and Government for my master's degree after I graduated from Tulane in 1967. I passed up admissions to the University of Pennsylvania and the University of Virginia to be closer to my family in New York. I secretly hoped I might repair the damage done with my dad's family so that I might have some normal relatives to share family time with.

In April 1968, my fellow Columbia grad students and I who were working on masters and doctorate degrees in political science were also attempting to figure out the different perspectives of reality held by the pro-Vietnam spokespeople and our campus anti-war protesters. The riots at Columbia had occurred that month, and we were sifting through the leaflets of the Students for a Democratic Society as well as absorbing the timeless wisdom of ancient philosophers. This time the synthesis we were attempting addressed the position of our nation's moral compass and value sets. We had hoped we might construct means by which both sides could engage in meaningful dialogue. Nevertheless, the elusive integration of political and moral polarities between pacifism and war eluded us, once again.

So did my hoped-for independence from my mother. I realized that my next step toward a separation from her smothering would be when I married, and I knew I had to choose a strong man who would not also be cowed by her outbursts and mental illnesses. I met that man in 1969.

CHAPTER THREE

Adult Lightning Strikes

My dearest friend from college, Celine Weinberg, often came up from Texas where she lived to visit her aunt Beverly, who lived in New Jersey. Celine's routine was to stay with her cousin, Richard "Rick," and his wife Glenda and their little girl Melissa. In the summer of 1969 her visit coincided with Rick and Glenda being secretly separated and nearing the end of divorce proceedings. Being the first couple to divorce in their respective families led them to hide the truth, so when Celine came to visit, Rick moved back in with Glenda and the charade began.

"Hey Rick," Celine segued during dinner about her graduate studies the first night of her visit, "I've gotta ask you if you have any friends down at the airport, maybe a private pilot like you, who'd like to ask out my best friend from college. She broke up with this guy after a year and she's kinda bummed out."

"Oh, I might know some guys," offered Rick, his interest piqued. Unbeknownst to her, he was considering me for himself. Except when he did call, the next day, he told me he was Richard Feldman's friend, and that his name was Rick Johnson. After three dates, we had both fallen in love, and he confessed his initial false persona to me.

I was over the moon. If I married Rick, I'd be the cousin of my dear friend, Celine. There was no way his introductory lie was going to spoil the romantic dreams I had begun to weave around the ideal life I would live. If all worked out, I would be a part of his normal, high-functioning, happy, family. I had ironically met Rick's mother Beverly before I met him. Beverly, Celine, and I had gone to a Broadway show on one of Celine's trips to New York in 1969. At the time Beverly had said to me, "Lynne Donna, I wish my son had met and married you instead of the shrew he has now."

As 1969 drew to a snowy conclusion, no one had any idea Rick and I were involved. The deliciousness of a secret affair came to an end one day before New Year's when Rick brought over his wash for his mother, Beverly, to do.

"Interesting pink panties you've taken to wearing, my dear," she snidely remarked as she threw my underwear at him.

It was time for Rick to sit his father and mother down to explain that he and Glenda were divorcing, he had rented his own apartment, and I was his new girlfriend. It was also time for me to tell Celine who her cousin Rick had "fixed me up with." Celine was not amused I was in love with her cousin, or that Rick and Glenda were divorcing.

"So you're a home wrecker, are you?" she snapped at me, which hurt like a slap across the face.

"Wait, Celine, you've got this all wrong. Rick was separated when you stayed with him last year, you just didn't know it."

"They didn't look separated, Lynne, they looked like quite the happy suburban couple. I can't believe you're involved with a married man. How sick." She wouldn't back down from the accusation.

Rick later explained to me that Celine's mother and father had recently split and Celine was bitter over what she perceived as her dad causing the divorce.

❧ ❧

Mom and dad flew up to meet my new love, my fiancé by then. We met at a steak house in Manhattan. As the evening progressed, it appeared mom was delighted a marriage would soon be on the calendar. Toward the end of this initial meeting, we hit a bump when mom told Rick he'd better call her "Mom" after our marriage. Rick made it equally clear he'd be calling her "Leah." When she didn't get the same compliant response from him I always lavished on her, her face grew cold and disapproving. It dawned on her finally that Rick was in love with me and not with her.

64

"How *could* you love a man who doesn't love *me*?" she screamed over the phone after she flew home. "You can't possibly marry someone like that. You *promised* that anyone you loved would have to love me, too."

I had no memory of making any such promise, but knowing how I caved to any entreaty of hers, it was possible I did make that commitment. It did not occur to me to push back against any such commitment, real or imagined.

"I'll talk to him, mom, but he's not much of a 'pro-mom' fellow. He's not that close to his own mother and I think she's fabulous." I had begun to idealize my future mother-in-law as the type of normal upper middle class Jewish woman I hoped to become. Rick seemed to hold himself at a distance from her, which I couldn't figure out.

I had come from a troubled family, grappling constantly with my mother's psychoses. All I wanted was a stable and happy marriage as I set out to start my own family. Perhaps that wish might be unattainable. Perhaps once I became a married woman myself, and with the backing and support of Beverly, I thought, I might gain some distance from my mother's pressure. Beverly was a strong woman who, although much shorter than me, could have passed for my mother. She had hazel eyes and dyed blond hair with an ample bosom and a nicely proportioned body. I fantasized what being reared by her might have been like, with people smiling at her and wanting to be her friend. I, certainly, would be her ally, even if it meant siding with her against my mother and even at times against my own husband. I failed to register the trap I was stumbling into with two women pressuring me to modulate my boyfriend's emotions toward them.

Rick and I sought to spend more time with one another and distance ourselves from the growing pressure of my mother on our relationship. We joined a U.S. senatorial campaign and worked together in the same office seven days a week for ten months in 1970. If our candidate Nelson Gross won, we'd both become senatorial staffers in Nelson's New Jersey home office. But he lost. By a huge, deafening margin.

After Election Day I stood in the unemployment line pondering my fate while I waited to register for the paltry sum I was to receive. I had an Ivy League education, a strong résumé, and no job. This was not shaping up to be the stable life that I wanted so desperately. How could I settle the ground under my feet?

I would create stability for myself, I decided, by working at a profession I had once scoffed at as being too routine: I'd get a teaching degree and share my knowledge of American social studies with high school students. With my test scores and background there was no education school that would deny me, but I chose a college near my apartment. I enrolled at once in a program that would quickly grant me teaching certification on top of the master's degree I already possessed. While I was studying to get my teaching degree, Rick's divorce became final in January 1971. We agreed to marry on August 8th of that year.

The morning of my wedding, as mom and dad and I set off to the country club, the three of us got into a terrible fight.

"Lynne Donna, did you see how the Feldmans had their own rehearsal dinner without even the decency of inviting you and daddy and me to it? How selfish! How dare they hold a dinner alone the night before their son's wedding to you?" she shrieked.

"Leah, Leah," sighed my father, "This wasn't really a rehearsal dinner. We didn't have a rehearsal! It was just a dinner for the Feldmans, and let's not fight on our way to our daughter's wedding."

"I won't be disrespected in this manner by their hoity-toity family that thinks they're too good for us!" screamed mom. She was gearing up for a huge blow-up, it seemed. Her feral glare targeted my dad. "You never have the guts to stand up for your wife, do you?" Then she aimed it at me in the back seat. "And Lynne Donna, what have you got to say for that man you're marrying? Can't you insist he respect your parents, or don't you care about us?"

She paused, and dad and I thought she might have run out of ammunition, but no, she was just taking a breath. "You know what old man Feldman [Rick's father] told me yesterday? 'It's too late to call off the wedding now, dearie.'" She imitated as snide an impression as she could muster with all of her dramatic flair.

I withheld the truth that Rick's family had already gotten wind of my mother and did not want to celebrate with her any more than they had to.

Arriving at the country club, I took my gorgeous lace wedding dress and tulle veil with shaking hands and legs and attempted to soothe myself by deep breathing before putting on my ceremonial attire.

Other than that, the wedding went off as I had hoped. I managed to ignore Mom's sulking over whatever slight she imagined she'd suffered during exchanges with the wedding guests or relatives. I had successfully married Rick (who was not a shoe salesman) in a beautiful ceremony without having gotten him to love my mother.

When we returned from our honeymoon, we took up residence in a house we built to our specifications. It was the house in the suburbs that I saw in my childhood dreams, with a huge expanse of forest behind it populated by quail, wild turkeys, skunks, and other delightful woodland creatures. I would have my teaching degree by May 1972 and could begin looking for a permanent position that summer. My best friend was now my cousin and I had married into my fantasy of a loving, extended family.

The first three months after our wedding appeared to be healing so many wounds. But after the three-month honeymoon period of our marriage, Rick and I discovered we had a similarly unfortunate theme running through our formative years: we had both been scapegoats. After our wedding, when everything looked so promising, I began to hear Beverly refer to Rick's younger sister, Jean, as the "good" and "perfect" child. My husband, on the other hand, was always referred to as the "bad" one or "black sheep." Other female family members validated this status among themselves and to me personally. I was reminded many times how "difficult" he was for Beverly when he was a child.

"Jean," Beverly bragged to me, "could be thrown down in her crib and she wouldn't bother me, but your husband, I could never break."

I was horrified a mother would rue the fact she had not "broken" one child, and brag about the other child who was far easier to "break".

Beverly's treatment of Rick, as he came to recall events of his childhood to me early in our marriage, was pretty grim. In one of many fits of rage, she threw a cooking kinife at young Rick that landed in his elbow. Instead of apologizing, she rationalized to him "it was the closest thing I could get my hands on." From his earliest recollection, Beverly continually threatened Rick with physical abandonment and being sent to live in a foster home. Throughout his life she humiliated him publically at every opportunity. When circled by family or friends, her tactic was to remark with Rick in earshot, "You wouldn't believe the stupid thing Rick did the other day." To his face and in front of family she would scold, "Why couldn't you be more like that nice young man Donny Levine?"

Rick and I began to share elements of our formative years together and indeed found a sad similarity in the psychological abuse with which we had both grown up. This unfortunate context bound us even closer together. Yet he tended to discount the pain caused by his parents' mistreatment. "So what?" he'd rationalize. "They gave me a roof over my head and three meals a day," he explained to me one night. "At least my parents weren't like your mother and her sisters who are just fucking nuts."

⁂

After our wedding my mother became desperate for Rick to cater to her every mood shift and weird demand as I did. In November 1971, she announced she, my dad, and their dog Lili were coming to visit right after we moved into our new home. This was fine with both of us, until she let slip she planned to stay for three months. She added that she was mailing seven cartons weighing between 40 and 50 pounds each containing her reference books, poetry, and art supplies. She told us she'd need them all during her prolonged stay. I felt trapped—my husband rightfully cried "foul" and demanded I tell her a week or two would be fine, but three months was a tenancy. This fell into a pattern during our first year of marriage: my mother would demand something outrageous from us; my husband would fume at top volume that the situation was intolerable; and I was caught in the middle.

"Whose side are you on?" my new husband barked at me about

their impending trip. "It had better be mine or we can end this marriage now. I'm calling my lawyer—you know, the same one I used to divorce Glenda."

I couldn't stand this broadside and screamed, "I'll do anything! Just tell me what I can do to save this marriage!"

The answer was obvious. "Stop this three-month visit!"

I called up my mother and, while crying, tried to get her to see what damage she was causing. "Mom, this could be the end of my marriage, and I love Rick. Please don't come up for three months—it isn't fair to us in our house that hasn't much furniture anyhow."

"Lynne Donna, you are being disrespectful to your mother and father," she responded sternly. "But if that man is so stubborn and hateful to your parents, then we will only stay for three weeks. That isn't what I hoped would happen, but so be it. You're at fault here for not fighting for your mother and father. Let it go at that."

With tears, lots more begging, and taking the blame for the "shortened" visit, I got my mother to agree to a three-week stay, which was miserable for us all in a three-bedroom split- level with little furniture. The good news during this fiasco of a visit was my receipt of a teaching contract at Central Valley High beginning September 5, 1972.

Once I began the job, I found it anything but routine. It turned out to be the perfect canvas for my quirky creativity. Colonial history led me to teach students how to quilt and churn butter; I turned the class into a replica of the United States Senate while studying the battle over secession of the Southern states in 1861, with each student playing the role of an actual senator from that time; and I escorted my students to model sessions of the United Nations and U.S. Congress at various academic venues around the east coast. I became a popular, honored, and well-respected teacher and was thrilled to go to work each day.

I had a theory that there were three parts to a life: professional, personal, and social. If I could keep at least one of them in perfect shape, then I had a fair shot at a stable life. Of course, the ideal was to get all three stable. But my personal life never seemed to reach a balance. My theory came from my childhood in which my mother made my life unstable on all three fronts. The woman I was looking to now was a person I hoped could guide me toward successful professional, personal, and social functioning.

On a trip to Florida in 1972, while Rick stood with his mother in the foyer about to exit their new condo, and with an absence of outward provocation, she suddenly balled her fists and began to beat him on the head for over a minute. I had never witnessed physical domestic violence before. I couldn't breathe and felt that old numbing sensation seep throughout my body. Rick stood still initially for the blows. I ran forward to grab his hand, and the two of us fled her apartment for our car. Once securely out of her reach, Rick acknowledged with hushed tone, "I think I was an abused child." It was at this point that stories of his abysmal childhood flooded back into his consciousness. Not only had he been psychologically abused throughout his life, but also both his mother and father had routinely beaten him. It was a memory and fact that would take him decades to process.

"My Jean is a perfect mother and wife," Beverly had bragged to me prior to her attack on Rick. Now that I was officially her daughter-in-law, Beverly became freer in her condemnation of Rick and her doubting of my capabilities as Melissa's stepmother. I fell into confusion and self-doubt as I saw my hopes for a role model turn on me and inflict physical and emotional pain on my husband. Why had I thought Beverly was so "perfect?" Was her lack of overt mental illness enough to fool me into thinking she was "the one" who could teach me what I was so hungry to learn about a good life?

Perhaps mental illness did follow me into my married extended family. Beverly had further grist for the mill in victimizing both Rick and me over Melissa, beginning when the child was three and she began violent behavior in her pre-school class. We kept Beverly and Jean from hearing about these serial episodes of Melissa's misconduct, hoping this was merely a phase she would grow out of, once she had metabolized her parents' divorce. When Melissa was reported to have poked her kindergarten classmates with sharp pencils, we kept the child's behavior secret from her aunt and grandmother lest they think ill of their little relative. But once Melissa was referred to a child psychiatrist, the family found out and sought to cast blame on us. We figured they must have projected the humiliation of having mental illness in their family on us as the agents of the problem. Did Melissa inherit mental issues from Beverly and her violent episode rather than from the divorce, I wondered? I began to doubt I had escaped anything by marrying into Rick's family; rather, it began to appear that I had married into a second hornet's nest.

Glenda refused to take Melissa to her psychiatric appointments, so Rick and I often were saddled with that chore. One psychiatrist complained to us that Glenda really wanted to have Melissa dropped off at her office, and for the doctor to parent Melissa instead. Shortly after we returned from the ill-fated trip to Florida where Rick's mother accosted him, Rick and Glenda were called to Melissa's kindergarten class for a discussion with her teacher and her principal over Melissa's overt acts of aggression against her classmates. Glenda was ill and would not go, so I went with Rick. When I entered the classroom, Rick got a cold glare, but hatred filled the principal's eyes when she saw me.

"You should be ashamed of yourself," the principal threw at me as I sat down in the pint-sized chairs. "I called you over and over to arrange a conference about your daughter's violent behavior, and you never bothered to respond to my calls. What kind of mother are you?" As a new teacher myself, I knew that such a blatant attack on me was both unprecedented and unprofessional, yet I was so taken aback that I remained silent until Rick burst out in my defense.

"Wait a minute," he forcefully interjected, "this isn't Melissa's mother, Glenda! This is Lynne, my new wife and Melissa's *step*mother. How dare you treat her that way?"

It is never easy to marry someone with a small child, and it is even harder with a man whose young daughter showed emotional shadows from the beginning. Glenda's domestic situation ensnared Melissa in an even more difficult life situation when Glenda was diagnosed with multiple sclerosis in 1972.

Right after her devastating diagnosis, Glenda married Herb Stern without sharing the fact of her illness with him. He was a new widower with two small children to raise. The mix of a disturbed child coming into a blended family dynamic was toxic and placed Melissa in the position of a scapegoat there as well.

In the summer of 1972, when school was out, Glenda called us to take Melissa for days at a time. "Herb and I are taking Dara and Peter to an amusement park, and Melissa shouldn't come. She'd just mess up our enjoyment." Leaving Melissa out of their family plans expanded to include dinners and visits to relatives that summer. Even Glenda's neighbors confided in us that neither she nor Herb were treating Melissa well.

Rick and I tried to weave Melissa into our family on her weekend stays and day visits as I was still attempting to create the happy, functional Jewish family I never had. I arranged all the religious and cultural rituals a Jewish wife is supposed to manage: Seders; observations of all major Jewish holidays; cooking a modified kosher diet; and learning the observances for weekly Sabbath meals.

While I was struggling to offer my husband's troubled daughter a safe, second home, I still had to deal with my mother. She presented me with her usual erratic behavior and hysterical demands and accusations. But I was growing numb to my mother's tirades as I now had my hands full with Melissa. My stress level began to hit lifetime highs over the growing rift between Melissa and her mother, and now the barrage of calls from my mom about her painful injury received aboard a cruise ship. It seems that the shower in her cabin misfired a burst of boiling water that scalded her hand. It had to be bandaged for weeks and was quite legitimately painful.

This combination of stressors, I believe, caused my immune system to become compromised and overwhelmed. Shortly after my mother's injury I came down with pneumonia and was over-prescribed tetracycline by my doctor. I broke out in plate-sized rashes that required hospitalization. This toxic medical reaction also resulted in a condition similar to rheumatoid arthritis, and I was sent home from work for two weeks to recuperate.

That summer of 1973, after I regained use of both hands without pain, Glenda started handing off Melissa to us even more frequently. I had more opportunities to observe the child's unstable behavior up close. She would suddenly start screaming and thrashing around violently. It was a long, slow, and difficult summer trying to be kind and patient with Melissa, but even harder to impose anything resembling discipline. Having grown up with a mentally ill and

72

unstable person constantly around me, this was all oddly familiar. It was as frustrating as dealing with my mother. I never knew how to curb her outbursts or soothe my mother, and the same proved true with Melissa.

Melissa entered second grade the following fall where her behavior continued to puzzle and upset all of us. Every day in school brought a different crisis. I was often called out of my class to go to Melissa's school to take her back to her mother's home, and I was beginning to get criticism from my supervisors for the absences. Tests indicated she had an above-average I.Q. and abilities. She was intelligent enough to get into and graduate from college but her emotional stability and behaviors were destructive to addressing traditional learning environments and tasks. The school special education team could not figure out sufficient techniques to moderate her outbursts.

By 1974 Melissa was suicidal, but we did not know this until she reported it to us as an adult. Her mother began to send her to us every weekend and most nights after school so she could mother "her other" children. Glenda and Herb mercilessly mocked Melissa by creating hurtful nicknames for her, or by calling attention to the fact that she had a last name different than theirs. Otherwise, she was a cute little brunette replica of her dad with curly thick hair and her grandmother Beverly's smile. She spent time reading in her room and sketching. But while with us, I couldn't control her behavior, which included cursing and throwing insults at adults as I held her hand walking through the mall. If only I could reach inside her troubled soul and have her receive the love that I tried to share with her, I naively believed that love was all she needed to "cure" her behavior. Rick became despondent over his daughter's behavior and would not honor discussions about perhaps starting our own family as I was turning twenty-nine.

With my mother writing me 10-page letters disparaging how little time I was devoting to her, I began slipping into depression. Our marriage was definitely damaged, and by the end of my parents' annual stay with us that winter, Rick and I wondered if our beautiful new house had become "haunted" by my mother. I could not erase the sense-memory of my mother sitting with me on the living room sofa on my 29th birthday and verbally abusing me.

"Lynne Donna, how could you permit that husband of yours to dictate when Daddy and I come up to visit you and how long we can stay? This is your home too, but he's the big boss and you seem to have nothing to say."

"Mom, on one visit you sent up your entire *Encyclopedia Britannica*, all of your oils and brushes and several canvases in addition to your poetry books," I reminded her. "How could we not think you were planning to move in for months?"

"I am your mother and I should be welcome to stay with my own daughter as long as I want. Besides, that Melissa gets her own bedroom. I don't see you showing her the same limits in your house as you put on Daddy and me. You're a shameful daughter! All I ever asked was that you have a husband who could love your mother and you can't even do that one simple thing for me. I hate to say this about my only child, but you are a complete disappointment."

"Mom," I responded with a mock smile that portrayed how disgusted I was with her, "Thanks for this discussion on my birthday. Now I want to put my head in the oven." I got up abruptly, went to my bedroom, slammed the door shut, threw myself across the bed, and buried my face in the pillows.

In 1977 when Melissa was ten, Glenda's multiple sclerosis became demonstrably worse, and their family decided to take a trip to Europe. We received a call from Glenda in Paris three weeks into their trip:

"This is no longer fair to my children and my husband. We can no longer stand Melissa's behavior, her screaming tantrums and rudeness." Her voice was full of frustration and she didn't pause for a breath. "As much as I'm concerned by what the neighbors will say about this, I'm sending her to live with you permanently." No discussion, just notice that Melissa was being flown home alone from Europe that day and we were to pick her up at the airport.

We embraced her and enrolled her in the local public school system that September. I wrote her funny little notes that I placed in her lunchbox every day. I introduced her to everyone as "my daughter" and I took over all of the nurturing and practical chores of a mom. But Melissa's disruptions showed up in the public school as soon as she was enrolled. On her first day at her new school, she angrily upended an entire shelf of books that scattered the length of the classroom and could have injured someone. We were called to a conference when she was found hiding in garbage cans instead of going to her class. Then came Back to School Night.

"Why are the parents glaring at us?" I whispered to Rick as we stood amidst student dioramas. We found out after the session when Mrs. Everly asked to speak with us.

"Mr. and Mrs. Feldman, I cannot have someone like Melissa in my class. She runs out of the room whenever she wants, taunts and shoves the other students, and is foul-mouthed. We need to speak with the superintendent about her presence in this school."

"I hope it doesn't have to come to that. Melissa has had emotional problems since her mother rejected her, and I'm sure that's why she's behaving the way she is," Rick tried explaining.

"I'm really not interested in an explanation, sir. I have twenty other well-behaved children who deserve an education that's not disrupted by one little girl."

Unbeknownst to us, a decision to expel her had already been reached. We were again on a search for a diagnosis and an appropriate venue for her education. The school system paid to have her transferred to a school where other children with behavior problems could receive therapy within an academic setting. Yet no satisfactory diagnosis could be found for Melissa's behavior. We heard depression, borderline psychotic, antisocial personality disorder, bipolar disorder, and several other guesses. Rick and I took her to psychiatrists in New Jersey and New York seeking answers. Melissa was getting sadder, angrier, and more destructive.

The special school for the emotionally disturbed was not able to curb her behavioral outbursts and aggressive behavior. There was no other school in a reasonable distance that could handle an acting-out female student. We found a military boarding school for her an hour away where we thought she might receive the means by which she could learn to control and curb her rages. But after a few months at the boarding school, the administration told us they could not handle such an ill child.

"I loved that school," sobbed Melissa when we came to pack up her trunk and once again remove her from a place she had come to trust. "And I was so good at close-order drill I won a commendation for my platoon." She sadly took off her uniform for the last time. She just couldn't help herself when she was misbehaving. Once she came home again, she was tutored for a few hours by teachers from the middle school while Rick drove her around the rest of the time as he went about his work. It wasn't an optimum situation for any of us.

During this time, I asked Rick once again if we could start our own family. I was Melissa's mother full-time now, and felt that it was only fair to have a baby of my own to love and nurture.

"I'm not keen to have another baby, hon," admitted Rick. "Look at the problems we're having with Melissa. Could you handle another baby with problems, either physical or mental? And is mental illness inheritable? Look at your mother and aunts. We'd be buried alive if we had two kids with issues. Having a baby is about the lowest item on my list of priorities," he whispered to me as we huddled in bed one night.

"But that's not fair!" I protested.

With the stress of dealing with Melissa's instability, our marriage was in trouble, but I still wanted a child of my own. "I shouldn't be punished for Melissa's illness. I want my own baby and it has just as much chance to be bright and normal as any other child."

"The odds aren't great," Rick replied. "Plus, what about Melissa's shrink? He warned us not to add a baby to the family as long as Melissa is having psychotic breaks and acting out."

These psychotic breaks took a variety of forms. Some consisted of screaming and thrashing about until physically restrained; others involved injuring herself; still other times her hygiene was compromised. She began distorting her life with us to her grandmother and relatives by reporting how terribly we were caring for her, and accused us of making her go without new clothes. On top of all of this, there was no place that would agree to school her.

In the spring of 1979, my immune system was once again fragile. I contracted pneumonia after a protracted asthmatic-bronchitis attack and was beginning to recover, but for a deep cough. My illnesses during Melissa's time with us became more frequent and virulent, as if my body were warning me that I had taken on far too much for my body to handle. I had no time to engage in any form of self-care, and was running myself ragged. I no longer had the strength to deal with her. My commitment, resolve, and techniques for stemming her outbursts had dwindled. Neither by adding structure nor by being loving and tolerant was I able to exact any aspect of non-threatening or controlled behavior. At one point I walked around the house with a clipboard and gave her stars whenever she acted normally. The stars could be redeemed for a treat, but this attempt at behavior modification failed too. I also tried spending what free time I had with her, taking her to horseback riding lessons, roller skating, and swimming, but nothing brought her to the point of bonding with me enough to stop her outbursts.

It was around this time that Melissa found a way to get me to my own breaking point. We had gotten into the car for her to be taken to her psychiatrist when she began ear-piercing screams as she told me how horrible I was as her mother. She wailed to the point of rattling my nerves, and I slapped her on her thigh hoping she'd stop. She didn't. I had never struck her before or again, but I saw how she could push me to my edge.

At my wit's end, I needed a weekend away just for me alone to clear my head during the summer of 1978. Rick arranged for me to visit with another cousin, the daughter of one of Beverly's favorite sisters, Ruth, and her family for that weekend. When Ruth asked me what was happening in my home, I could not bring myself to tell her the extent of Melissa's illness or how bizarre her behaviors were. I reported only the least objectionable of her behaviors. My lack of being truthful and specific about the very serious nature of her behavior led them to discount how dire the situation truly was. Ruth saw me off at the airport as I returned home and summed up her thoughts: "Melissa is just a poor kid who's been bounced around too much by her parents. Make sure you give her good, loving parenting."

But Rick and I later learned that Beverly and Jean had a conversation after my visit with Ruth. Jean and her husband then called Rick and suggested they raise Melissa along with their three children. Beverly spoke to both Rick and me about the possibility of a switch in unofficial custody the next day.

"Look, you two, neither of you can hold a candle to Jean as a mother with her three perfect children. Jean could have done, and will do, a better job at raising Melissa as one of her happy three children. Admit it; you've both failed as parents."

"Go to hell!" responded Rick. It would be the last time mother and son spoke.

Melissa went with her little suitcase packed almost as it had been after being sent home from Paris by her mother and the military boarding school. There were only losers in this arrangement, and Jean came next.

CHAPTER FOUR

Melissa

Over the next three weeks, all we heard were calls from Melissa telling us how wonderful life was with Jean, and how she and her three cousins adored each other. Melissa met up with Rick's other cousins and their children, who felt sorry for the poor little girl who was so badly treated by her stepmother and father. She bragged about how they all loved her and invited her to their parties and celebrations, a family inclusion I had so longed for myself and for my children when they came along.

As much as it wounded our egos that Jean was apparently raising Melissa better than we had managed, we dared to dream that this situation might become permanent and we could breathe normally in our home. Three weeks with Melissa at Jean's, and with our household limping back to a quiet normal rhythm, I felt reborn, and Rick began to regain his sense of humor. But a week later we received a hysterical call from Jean. It turned out things had actually not been going well from the very beginning.

"You ruined this child! Even I can't raise her!" Jean shouted into the phone. "She's out of control, speaks dirty and crudely to me and my children, and can't get along with any of us. Expect her back on tonight's plane from Ithaca. I'm washing my hands of this. Damn you both!"

After Rick went to the airport to claim his twelve-year-old being shuttled back and forth between homes and schools, Melissa entered the house as if nothing much had happened. "What's for dinner?" she asked as she threw down her suitcase.

Exhausted, Rick and I took Melissa to Florida over Christmas with us and left her off at Beverly's so we could enjoy a week's rest. We took time out to be a couple again, and by our return from winter break, I was pregnant. Rick was moderately enthusiastic, but held himself apart from me during the pregnancy, so fearful was he that we would produce a mentally or physically challenged child.

Melissa was furious that a baby was coming, and would sit at my feet as I knitted baby blankets chanting, "I hope the baby dies. I hope the baby dies. I hope the baby dies..."

My parents couldn't believe their great fortune to finally have one grandchild while they were still alive, and my mother painted the most gorgeous oils for me to hang in my little baby's room. I'd never seen her so happy. Beverly let me know that with four grand-daughters she was only interested if I had a son. It turned out I was carrying a daughter, and that was the end of the excitement over my pregnancy from Beverly.

Our daughter Erica Leigh was born in September 1979. Erica arrived with the dark brown eyes of her father, copper-colored curly hair that eventually hung in Shirley Temple ringlets, and two huge dimples just like Aunt Debbie's. She came into the world happy, compliant, and easy-going. *Boy, this is a breeze*, I thought to my-self. But then I encountered the challenge of keeping the baby safe around her half-sibling.

Melissa continued her screaming and thrashing behavior. At the first sign of one of these outbursts, Rick would physically move Melissa to the kitchen and close both doors, while I hurried Erica to my bedroom at the far side of our three-level home. I'd turn on music or begin to sing to my baby to distract her from the screams coming from the floor below. As Melissa's teeth chattered and she shook from inner demons, Rick would try his best to calm her down.

I was happy I had taken the entire academic year of 1979 to 1980 off for maternity leave so I could be with my beloved child and monitor Melissa's conduct around Erica. When I could find a baby-sitter, the woman would refuse to return unless Melissa was out of the house. I thus had the sole responsibility of monitoring Melissa's whereabouts at all times.

Melissa wasn't in school and was mostly driving around in the car with her father during the day. If he couldn't watch her, then wherever Melissa had to go, I had to take Erica, and vice-versa. Car trips were particularly intense: once strapped into our seats, Melissa would pick a fight and begin to shriek or cry, which then caused Erica to scream. From a happy little pumpkin, Erica began to get nervous to the point of recoiling around any loud noises.

I returned, quite reluctantly, to my teaching position in September 1980, just as Erica was about to turn one. I arranged for Erica to be watched by a wonderfully loving sitter, Susan, who often brought her teenage daughter, Susanna, to play with Erica, which was an ideal situation for my little baby. They were joined on weekends by their friend, Sister Anne, who worked at the local monastery. As Erica grew into a little toddler she often went to play at the monastery and became a favorite of Father Rocco, which tickled all of us to see this interfaith crew with habits, collars, rompers, and shorts cavorting on swings and slides. Susan did not associate with Melissa and was instructed to devote herself to Erica, so the situation hobbled along at home. I tried leaving school quickly each day so I might give Susan as little time as possible to be alone with Melissa. I couldn't be on top of her every second and when she wasn't hurting those around her, she found ways to hurt herself.

⚮

I returned to class that fall but repeatedly received calls to come claim Melissa wherever she happened to be. Her language was foul and aimed at everyone within hearing range. No one had any idea how to curb her tongue or her behavior. This was one desperately unhappy child who was taking out her frustration on all those around her. A major source of Melissa's anger came from being rejected by her mother, Glenda, who restricted Melissa's visits to her home on Long Island. These visits became briefer and briefer.

She called me "mom" or "ma" by then too, since I was now her primary caretaker. Being identified as her mother earned me nasty glares from women in the malls and restaurants when she screamed or yelled insults at passersby. Yet I could not forbid Melissa the security of calling me her mother since her own had basically abandoned her, even if I was mistaken for a terrible mother with an out-of-control child.

One of the saddest and more upsetting exchanges I had with Melissa involved her growing estrangement from her mother. On a chilly fall day in 1981, Melissa and I were playing with Erica on the floor of her bedroom with large cardboard blocks that we could build into chairs and fortresses. My attention was focused on how to create a tunnel through which Erica might crawl, when Melissa brought up the subject of adoption.

"Ma, I have to tell you. I watch how you love and care for Erica and I think you are the best mother I've ever seen. Would you please adopt me right away so I could be your real child?"

My glance swiveled over to her face to see if she was being sincere with me; her face showed no duplicity or contempt. I was startled and stymied. How was I to answer her? I was actually tempted to say "Yes" because I knew it would add to her sense of having a foundation upon which to build her life. But I knew by then that mentally ill people had a toxic effect on me. I couldn't handle my mother or her sisters or Melissa herself, and I felt profoundly guilty that I didn't have more patience or unconditional love to give them. I also knew that I didn't love her the way I adored Erica. This wouldn't be an answer for either of us.

I took a long breath to give me a few moments to compose a loving but honest answer before I began speaking. "Melissa, honey, thank you so much for the nice things you just said to me. I'm really honored that you'd like me to be your real mom, but sweetie, you have a real mom already. I know things are rough right now between you two, but they can always get better, and your mom never, ever, suggested she would give you up as her daughter, just that it was better that you come to live with daddy and me."

I thought I had done a fair job of explaining why I could not honor her desire. But she had been thinking about this strategically and continued with her thoughts on the matter.

"Mom, I've thought about that. I do have a real mom, a birth mom, but you know what? If you can't adopt me, then I want to go back and live with my real mom. And if I hurt Erica, did something

82

really bad to her, then you and daddy would have to send me back to my mother and she'd have to take me back. So that's what I've been thinking about. What do you think?"

"Oh, Sweetie," I held onto my sanity at this critical moment, but all I wanted to do was take my little cherub and flee my own home to a refuge away from anyone who might think of harming her. "I'm sure you know that isn't an answer. You wouldn't want to hurt Erica, would you?"

"Hey, I figured out how to make that tunnel!" she responded as a way of shutting off the enormity of the conversation she had started. I let the heaviness of our conversation settle by joining the tunnel project.

Later that day I told my mother about my conversation with Melissa and about her request for me to adopt her, but I left out the part about Melissa thinking of hurting Erica. Mom had a definite opinion about me and my likely response.

"I know you quite well, Lynne Donna, and you're too soft, not resolute enough, to say 'no' to that child. If you ever even consider adopting her, it will be the biggest mistake of your life and I won't speak to you again!"

It looked as though Melissa would be in our home unofficially forever, since Glenda never relinquished legal custody, and I had decided not to pursue the discussion of adoption. If I couldn't handle my own mother and aunts, how was I to handle a mentally ill teenager along with them, a baby, and a husband working two jobs?

In the late winter of 1982, when Melissa was still fourteen, her mother finally and begrudgingly permitted Melissa to spend the weekend with her, since Glenda's husband and stepchildren would be away visiting their relatives. Upon Melissa's return, she asked to speak to me while I was cradling Erica, who was feverish from bronchitis.

"Mom, I have to tell you something."

"Sure, honey, you can tell me anything that happened this weekend. How'd it go?"

"Mom, I stood over my mother most of the night holding a knife over her chest. It took all I could do not to plunge it into her heart."

After hearing this dire news, I remember shaking so strongly that I awoke Erica, sleeping in my arms. I steadied myself after placing my daughter in her crib, long enough to call Melissa's psychiatrist for help.

"You are to admit her to a mental hospital right after we hang up, or do not ever call me again," directed Dr. Martin, leaving no room for discussion.

The healthy part of Melissa, the brave and resilient part of her borderline personality, had cried out for help. It stopped her from committing an unspeakable act. In the end, Melissa agreed with Dr. Martin, so Rick and Glenda reluctantly agreed to place her in a residential mental hospital. It would take decades for us to heal from this episode.

Melissa went to a children's psychiatric hospital in New York where she still had legal residence. Her admitting psychiatrist at the time, Dr. Smithline, was a tall, ramrod-straight man with thinning hair and cool blue eyes. But he radiated professionalism and an aura of expertise about the difficult world of mental illness. Rick had kissed Melissa goodbye as she entered the anteroom to the locked ward; she looked relieved to be there.

We went to his office and as we sat down, he informed us, "I am so very sorry you had to take her into your home as you did. She should have been institutionalized when she was seven. Borderline psychotics wreak havoc on households and in mental institutions. It's a serious illness marked by unstable moods, behavior, and relationships."

"Why did she almost stab her mother?" interrupted Rick. He wasn't in the mood for a psychiatric lecture.

"Melissa's brief psychotic episodes put her at the severe end of the diagnosis."

I was once again too stunned to talk. I turned rigid and felt chilled as if part of myself left my body, and I began to shake violently. I hugged myself as best I could, and I let Rick continue to lead the discussion.

"Doctor, why does she have these extreme reactions to everything? First she told my wife what a perfect mother she was, and a day later screamed at Lynne in the car that she was the worst mother and Melissa hated her."

"Rick, you've described the borderline personality perfectly. There's also another component to their behavior that we call the 'let's you and him fight' dynamic."

"I'm not sure what you mean, Doctor." Rick was doing the talking, but he was echoing my own puzzlement at the terms and phrases the psychiatrist was using.

"It's something borderlines do to set the people around them against each other. They consciously create splits in those around them, conflicts that put them in the center of attention and the other two parties angry with one another. I've already alerted the staff that we have a borderline coming into the ward. She'll try to create tension and fights between the staff, medical personnel, and other patients."

Rick and I looked at each other, uncertain what to do or say next. The doctor spoke a bit more, but his words just floated around the room. I recalled my father checking my mother into hospitals and thought I should be better equipped to handle this, but I wasn't.

After we left Melissa in the psych ward, Rick and I drove for an hour and a half across Long Island to New Jersey in frozen silence. Rick had just permitted his fourteen-year-old daughter to check herself into a locked mental facility. Glenda was only concerned about which insurance would be used for the stay.

"Did I do the right thing, hon?" he asked me as we entered our home without Melissa. "Did I have any other choice than to agree to let Melissa enter a mental ward?"

I hugged him with all my strength, and assured him that he had done the right thing. Hadn't my dad felt the same way when he entered my mom into a sanitarium? Didn't he chastise himself about how effective her treatment might be? The families of mentally ill patients share in the same terrible anxiety and self-doubt as the patients.

Next, the doctor met with Beverly and Jean who flew in that same week to find out why Melissa needed to be placed in a locked psychiatric facility.

"May I speak with you next week in person, Mr. Feldman?" the doctor asked shortly after Beverly and Jean departed. "I had a very unpleasant discussion with your relatives. And please bring your wife. She's involved in this as well."

I was terrified when the appointed time arrived. I had been demeaned unfairly before, and now there was the possibility that I would be scapegoated again. The message he gave us made me feel hopeless before I even arrived. Seated once again in his office, the doctor launched into what happened during Beverly and Jean's visit.

"Mr. and Mrs. Feldman let me first tell you how sorry I am about what I'm going to say." I began to focus intently on the doctor's words.

"I explained to your mother and sister very carefully that neither of you had any role in Melissa's profound illness. If Queen Elizabeth herself had raised Melissa, she'd have still turned out this way. But they couldn't hear me correctly and were receiving what I was telling them on a two-year-old's cognitive level."

"I'm sorry, Doctor," Rick interrupted, "I don't understand what that means."

"The best way to explain it is how toddlers don't know the difference between fantasy and reality. I'm so sorry to tell you that regardless of how strongly I tried to explain your lack of responsibility for Melissa's condition, they were firm in holding onto blaming you both."

"But didn't you explain what you told us? What did they say when you told them neither of us made Melissa ill?"

"They refused to hear what I had to say and just argued with me. Melissa is a borderline personality with psychotic episodes, and her behavior fits right into the criteria. You did nothing to provoke any of her behaviors."

"Is there any hope of reconciliation with my mother and sister based on what you've seen?" Rick asked plaintively, like a small boy.

The doctor stared at his folded hands on his desk. He avoided Rick's eyes, but finally looked up and said, "I never give up hope, but based on what I've seen, it will be close to impossible."

My world crashed down upon me in the hospital. There was nowhere to flee for safety. My dreams once again had disintegrated within a cauldron of mental illness, this time my stepdaughter's. My mother and her sisters stole my childhood, and now this fourteen-year-old child's illness had seeped into my adult life and what I hoped might be a substitute for the crazy family life I had grown up with.

After my second visit with the doctor at the mental hospital when we discussed Beverly's and Jean's visit, I could not bear to see Melissa in a locked mental ward. Despite the professionalism at this children's psychiatric hospital, the place filled me with the same fear and terror I felt as a young child when mom returned from treatments. Repetition made my fearful reactions more extreme, not less.

Although we were assured by all her psychiatrists that neither Rick nor I could possibly be the cause of Melissa's illness, Jean and Beverly laid complete blame at our feet and so informed their entire family, including my close friend, Celine.

One call from Celine shortly after Melissa's hospitalization sent me into a stark depression where I actually thought of giving up my beloved child.

"Lynne," Celine began, "you are the worst person in the world. I have no idea why I'm talking to you."

Once again I was taken completely aback and unprepared to defend myself against a strong personal attack.

"What on earth are you talking about, Celine?" I gagged at her cold words.

"You know goddamn well what I am referring to, you *horrible* person! You kept Melissa in your basement and you refused to feed her or buy her clothes. You don't deserve that gorgeous baby of yours," she snarled.

"Wait a second, Celine, we don't even have a basement..." I began, only to hear the phone slam down. I called her back immediately to try to explain that none of what she was reporting was true, but she kept to her assertion that I had treated Melissa with extraordinary cruelty and neglect. Beverly had done her best to demonize me to the entire extended family, it seemed.

I realize in hindsight that I should have been receiving counseling during this critical period, but I associated mental health workers with only the most disturbed individuals, and I was outwardly handling this chaotic situation with aplomb while succeeding in my career. This left me with no one to help me combat the scapegoating.

Rick's mother went so far as to encourage her extensive family of brothers, sisters, and cousins to cease acknowledging Erica's existence. She called me that year with a growling tone in her voice: "You've ruined my family. You think you're so *noble*." She exaggerated the word in an up-and-down singsong that dripped with sarcasm.

"What is that supposed to mean?" I tried to get clarity on what she thought I had done that was so damnable, but she hung up on me, and we never spoke again.

In response to these acts by his mother and the rest of her family, Rick decided to "divorce" his family by changing his name in 1985, and by Erica and me assuming his new last name as well. Although the memory of his abandonment and victimization did not cease, his anger subsided. This change of legal identity was a saving grace for him, and during a Chinese dinner one night we figured out what his new name should be. He left behind the victimized "Richard Harold Feldman" and became "Eric Harrison Fields."

Beverly's selection of Rick as a victim stemmed back to marital discord that started after Rick was born. She once told me, "Rick cried from his eczema so much as a newborn that my husband threatened to leave me. I couldn't keep that kid quiet." Her other remarks to me about her only son reflected this impression that somehow Rick's very existence was an affront to her.

Melissa was released from the locked ward at the mental hospital after a year and went into a residential treatment center in Westchester County. About this time, a distant relative informed Rick that his father was dying. Beverly continued her rejection of her son by refusing to let Rick know where his dad was hospitalized so the two men might say their final goodbyes. Beverly then instructed the family not to inform Rick when his father finally passed. No notice was given to us about his funeral or burial.

Only years later did a sympathetic relative let Rick know where his father had been buried so he could visit the grave. Rick felt terrible that he had been robbed of the opportunity to give his final loving respects to his dad. Our extended family was quickly shrinking with many relatives no longer speaking to us, and now his dad had passed away

CHAPTER FIVE

Law, Disorder, and Integral Theory

By 1982, Rick made it clear we were not going to have any more children. Our family would remain tiny.

"How can you even imagine bringing another child into this mess?" he spoke with annoyance. "We've got one child who's been in a mental hospital, another who's a perfectly behaved little girl. And you want to roll the dice and maybe get a version of your mother or aunts? No way. We have two children and that's going to be it. It's costing us for both of them and I can't afford another child."

I desperately wanted another baby and a sibling for Erica, but Rick had closed the door. Soon thereafter, the school where I taught figuratively closed its doors on me. In 1982, Central Valley's high school population dwindled from 1,400 to 660 students. I was given my layoff notice in April. "I don't want anyone to have control over when I'm working, ever again," I reasoned, and then countered Rick, "If there isn't going to be another baby, I'm applying to law school. I've wanted to do that since high school. It's the perfect next career for me."

It was more than wish fulfillment; it gave me an opening to a transformed life and hours away from domestic tension at night. I'd be able to play with Erica all day and then I'd be off in night class or staying late at the library. More importantly, I had wanted to be a lawyer since I was fifteen, but in the South in the 1950s and 1960s, this was a difficult path for a female. After I graduated from Tulane in 1967, I had taken the law school admission test (LSAT) and done well, yet when I spoke to several women lawyers in New Orleans, they discouraged me from choosing such a chauvinistic career path. But by 1982, the culture was far more accommodating and women made up nearly half of the graduating class.

"How can you do law school with a toddler at home? Won't it cost double for classes plus care for Erica? We just can't afford it all," responded Rick with a severe frown.

"Look, hon, law school is an investment in a lifetime career for me. Whether I work for a large firm or am self-employed, I can always be the master of my own destiny rather than wait for a pink slip from a school." This argument persuaded him that we could pay for law school plus hire someone to watch Erica while I was in class.

I took the LSAT, where I scored near the top, and with my high GPAs from Tulane and Columbia, I was told I could shoot for the moon—any law school would admit me. But I had a baby at home; Columbia did not have a night division; New York University was too far away for me to travel on a nightly basis; and I didn't want to travel to Newark, which was still a dangerous city back then. Eventually, I settled on Pace Law School in White Plains, New York. I was admitted immediately, and began classes on August 18, 1982.

Attending law school at night gave me a challenging schedule. I awoke at 8:00 A.M. every day to take Erica to nursery school, play dates or doctors' appointments. Susan, my sitter, arrived at 4:30 P.M. so that I could drive my clunky diesel car to White Plains and be in class from 6:00 to 10:00 P.M. four nights a week for four years. I would return after 11:00 P.M., and Rick would get home from his second job after midnight. After catching up with the events of his day, I would study and do my assignments for the next day's classes until 4:00 or 5:00 A.M., sleep until 8:00 A.M., and then awaken Erica to begin our day again. Four hours of sleep a night put additional stress on my body, and that was followed by spending the weekends in the law library doing research on LexisNexis, one of the few legal research computers available to us.

Over the years, I had never given up my search for a synthesis of polarities, the black or white questions that hung over issues such as science and religion, conservatism and liberalism, autonomy and community, or war and peace. Long before the advent of the Internet, I raced through journals looking for the key word "synthesis."

Finally, in 1982, I discovered the writings of Ken Wilber. I bought one of his few available books, and fell under the spell of his prose while studying for my law school finals. Specifically, I found myself aligned with his Integral Theory, and I saw how it could be used to discern differences and similarities between ostensibly remote fields of human discourse.

I discovered Wilber's work in a most curious manner. As I was sitting in the law library one weekend doing research for my torts paper, some student had left his copy of *Psychology Today* in the study carrel where I happened to be working. I had established a 45-minute rule for myself: after that length of research and writing, I'd take a fifteen-minute break by reading something light, so at the assigned break time I grabbed the magazine rather than the murder mystery I had brought along. Shuffling through the pages, I came across a full-page color photo of a lanky fellow with a bald head and mischievous smile. His name was Ken Wilber and the article described his emerging theory, which appeared to be the long sought after synthesis I had been investigating. I went directly to the bookstore the following day and ordered his book, *The Atman Project*, which I devoured in between briefing my legal cases.

Wilber helped me identify my mother's "either/or" and "us versus them" style of viewing the world as "dualistic thinking," where the world is divided into two opposing and never-to-be integrated parts. His work shone the light of clarity on her confusing logic. Her magic and mythic beliefs that her family members (and all Jews) were all good and blameless people exhibited a low level of sophistication and understanding of the world. This lower level of awareness he categorized as *pre-rational functioning*.

But Wilber also accommodated my mother's equally puzzling ability to tap into the highest spiritual and creative realms at times, the *trans-rational* realm, or that which is beyond the normal and rational abilities demonstrated by humans. Integral Theory thus initiated a complex and lifelong attempt to tease apart these disparate parts of my mother's character, and helped me make sense of my lived experience.

In the prologue to *The Atman Project*, Wilber states:

Everywhere we look in nature, said the philosopher Jan Smuts, we see nothing but *wholes*. And not just simple wholes, but hierarchical ones: each whole is a part of a larger whole which is itself a part of a larger whole. Fields within fields within fields, stretching through the cosmos, interlacing each and every thing with each and every other. (1979, p. 69)

To say this was a catharsis is an understatement: I nearly burst with understanding as I confirmed how my mother had developed unequally, and then proceeded to see where I fit into hierarchical development. Rather than feeling less sophisticated than others who were more highly developed consciously, I saw that my birthright was to develop as highly as I could. Wilber even set forth how it might be possible for me to pass from a less embracing awareness and consciousness to the next.

He also introduced me to the importance of understanding the difference between a translational perspective and a transformational one. Several of my acquaintances were engaged with teachers and gurus who were preaching transformation, but I wasn't at all sure what that meant, or how one achieved it. His simple explanation was that moving furniture around on the fourth floor constituted translation, but moving the furniture up to the seventh floor was transformation. There may come a time in my life when rearranging what I saw and how I was conscious of it was no longer satisfactory, and I would have to do the work of shifting to an entirely new way of seeing things. For the first time I began to feel optimistic about my future. If bad things happened to me, perhaps I might have better awareness of what caused the events rather than believing in the infantile curse of my mom's family.

Wilber even included an explanation as to why people like my mother, her family, and I had such unequal of levels of conscious development with many pre-rational yet also many trans-rational states:

[R]epression is one type of *failure* to cleanly transform (there are also arrest, fixation, dissociation, and regression). Should the self, in the process of transforming…encounter severe repression of, for example, aggression, then the ascent of consciousness is halted with regard to that facet of self. Or rather, from that stage on, the anger impulse will be *mis*-translated…. Thus transformation upward is distorted because, *at every stage* past the repression, the impulse is mistranslated….and these symbols represent the hidden aspects of self which now remain lodged in the lower levels of her own being. (1979, p. 117)

I could understand now why I never showed aggression toward my mother or her sisters.

I was hooked on Integral Theory, using it to work with myself, my family, and my legal studies. Yet where might I find a program that would synthesize the volumes of Wilber's work that I began to accumulate and translate? I begged my legal colleagues to discuss integral with me, but none of them had heard of Wilber or Integral Theory, so working with it on a personal level became a lone project for decades.

⚯⸱⸱⚯

The more I read Wilber, the more I wished he had created a user-friendly program by which I might understand the entirety of my life. How was I to fit in my marital discord, the mental illness within my family, and my need for a spiritual practice? I wanted anything by which I could find answers to my severe problems. I had my future law practice to nurture in addition to overseeing my father's and Aunt Ree's decline in physical functioning, and my grueling schedule in law school. In addition, I was Erica's Brownie Scout co-leader, the storytelling mom for her class, the Green Circle program presenter in the middle school, and a board member of our local tennis and swim club. I had to do it all, to feel that I deserved to be alive; I felt I had to pay some heavy dues to justify my space here, alive in human form.

In December 1985, I was deep into research for moot court competition in law school. I needed someone to watch Erica during the days before my babysitter came at 4:30 P.M. to take over. I recruited my parents for that winter break so I could devote myself to working at the law library for hours at a time studying for finals and preparing for moot court.

Moot court was a time I knew I would shine. With my acting experience and ten years of teaching, I felt at ease with the concept of battling my student adversaries before three actual judges. My partner, who took over half of the case we were assigned, was a beautiful marketing manager named Christie Jules. She assured me that she, too, felt at ease before large groups even if they were being hostile, as our adversaries would be. But I still felt obliged to remind her that legal argumentation cannot be handled as one does a promotional pitch that can be extemporaneously delivered. The facts had to be precisely recited and concepts deeply understood.

However, once my co-counsel began, it was apparent she wasn't prepared. Upon approaching the podium before the full auditorium, which was outfitted like a courtroom, Christie fainted dead away, and had to be literally dragged across the floor into the other room to be revived.

I felt badly for her but was not too alarmed until one of the three actual judges turned to me and said, "Well, Mrs. Feldman, you may go ahead and present both sides of your case, since surely as co-counsel you are as familiar with Ms. Jules' case as your own."

It was my turn to nearly faint, as I grabbed Christie's papers from the podium and made a game attempt to battle with her adversary while answering the judges' interjections. I did much better when permitted to handle my part of the argument, and won the American Jurisprudence prize for my efforts.

After that, when my parents returned to their home, tension arose to a fever pitch between me and my mother. She had witnessed Erica's energetic presence and decided her granddaughter was hyperactive and needed medical intervention. Seeing as I was overly obedient as a child, I realized that Erica's exuberance would have appeared negative to my mother, but I couldn't convince her otherwise.

"Lynne Donna, you have a disobedient child who won't sit still when you tell her to do so. She needs a firmer hand, which you obviously can't give her. I always thought you were too weak around your husband, and now I see you're too weak to discipline your daughter, too."

My pressure began to rise as I heard the caustic and condemnatory tone in her phone voice. "Mom, let's let this drop. I'll ask her pediatrician if he thinks she needs medication, but I'm telling you, she's fine, just nervous around Melissa when she goes into a tantrum."

"And that's another thing. You're permitting Melissa to ruin your daughter when she visits. Tell Rick he has to be stronger in disciplining them both."

I had had enough criticism. I decided to stop speaking to mom for a few months, but she continued to tell me my faults as a parent and human via ten-page letters once a week. I read them at first, but grew so depressed reading her negative views that I began to burn each one upon arrival, unopened, in my fireplace. I did not miss her presence during those months, and at least we were holding one mother at bay.

Neither Rick nor I had heard from his own mother, Beverly, since 1982. In 1985, Rick received a phone call from a close relative.

"Rick, your mother is dying in Florida and she demands you come to visit her before she dies. She's your mother and she deserves respect, even though you failed to give it to her all her life."

Rick was taken aback by his relative's call, the news about his mother, and the "demand" that after all of these years, he was expected to pay obeisance to his mother. A quick thinker, he responded, "Tell you what. When my mother can acknowledge to me that she has another granddaughter named Erica, I'll come down to be by her bedside."

She slammed the phone down, and he never heard from either of them again. But when he received news from his aunt that his mother had died, the aunt instructed Rick not to come to the funeral "because you'll make the occasion sad."

"What?" asked Rick, not sure he had heard correctly.

She repeated her warning, but at the end, Rick defied the lifetime of abuse and discord, and showed up at his mother's funeral to pay his final respects.

By 1986 I had my J.D., passed the bar on the first attempt, and demonstrated a talent for litigation. My mother and her sisters remained irritants, but a new chapter of my life was ready to unfold. As tentative and hesitant as I was in drawing boundaries with my mother, I was the reverse in court. Here was a safe venue for me to shine, to let out my assertive side with appropriate rules to keep either me or my adversary from stepping over the line into aggression.

My first-ever case as an attorney was a death penalty case, the *State v. William Bowlbey*, where I was chosen as co-defense attorney in 1987 literally a week after I was sworn in as a lawyer. Will, as he preferred to be called, was a young man who had been indicted for the strangulation with a broom handle of his 86-year-old neighbor. Will was a strange character: poised and gentlemanly with a British accent at times, he would promptly switch to ghetto-hoodlum speech and swagger. Was he a borderline psychotic, too? I couldn't figure him out, but without asking him directly if he killed his neighbor, my co-counsel and lead attorney Robert Gernsey and I considered Will to be highly dangerous and mentally unstable. Rob and I decided that my experience with my mentally ill mother, her sisters, and my stepdaughter made me the ideal person to handle Will, and it was I who spoke with him and prepped him for trial.

It took a year of pre-trial motions and case organization to get the case into court, and then a month to choose a jury that was prepared, if necessary, to impose the death penalty on our 29-year-old defendant. New Jersey still had the death penalty at the time, and its determination occurred after a defendant was found guilty of first-degree murder with aggravating circumstances. My deal with Gernsey, as we called him, was that I, as a brand new lawyer but experienced researcher and writer, would do all the research for, and writing of, the legal briefs that challenged different parts of the investigation and arrest. I would organize the 2,000 pages of discovery and be a great right-hand assistant to Gernsey when he handled the actual trial phase. This was in the pre-computer era, and it took me months to do the appropriate research and writing.

After a two-month long trial, our client was found guilty of first-degree murder with aggravating circumstances after 45 minutes of jury deliberation. Gernsey and I were horrified. We decided to go to lunch separately to lick our wounds before we returned to court to discuss with the judge and prosecutor how we would handle the penalty phase. But when Gernsey didn't show up at our meeting in the judge's office, I fled to the phone banks in the hall and called Belinda, our secretary.

"Belinda, this is Lynne. Look, this is urgent. Where the hell is Gernsey? He's nowhere to be found."

"Lynne, I can't bear to tell you this," she stammered. "He came in after the guilty verdict, threw his file on the floor, changed into his motorcycle gear, and left on his Harley straight out of town. We haven't seen or heard from him since!"

"What the hell do I do now? The judge and prosecutor are waiting for me in the judge's chambers to prepare for the penalty phase. I don't even know how that works!"

"I have no idea how to advise you, Lynne, Just go with whatever they tell you to do."

I returned to the judge's chambers with my head buzzing with scenarios that might mollify the others when I told them what was occurring, or what was not about to occur.

"Your Honor," I began, "Mr. Gernsey will not be joining us today, and I do not know where he is."

Judge Kiecken and the prosecutor, Jerry Gallo, immediately stood up. Their words were a blur in my consciousness. After they vented their outrage over Gernsey, they resumed their seats.

"Let this go on the record," intoned the judge. "Mr. Gernsey is not present today nor will he be. Co-counsel Lynne Feldman will be replacing him and will begin the penalty phase at 9:00 A.M. Monday morning."

"Wait a minute, Judge!" I interrupted with a frantic tone. "I've never even done a traffic ticket. How can Your Honor presume I can take over the penalty phase Monday?"

"Mrs. Feldman," the judge addressed me sternly as the court reporter clacked away making her official record of this fiasco. "Are you an attorney licensed to practice law in the state of New Jersey?"

"Yes, Your Honor, but—"

Now it was the judge who interrupted me.

"And therefore you are qualified under the laws of New Jersey and the United States Constitution to represent your client in court beginning this Monday at 9:00 A.M. This hearing is adjourned until then."

He abruptly rose and left for his private chambers, leaving the prosecutor and me slack-jawed.

Thus it was left to me alone, a newly admitted lawyer with not one minute of trial time under my belt, to plead for the life of my newly convicted client. Unfortunately, I cannot go into details of this chaotic situation because of attorney-client privilege, but things got even stranger. I wondered if I'd better hold onto Will's hands during the pronouncement of sentence to make sure he did nothing rash in court if the jury gave him the death sentence.

It was the Wednesday before Good Friday when I found out I would have to handle the case alone. The prosecutor informed me I had to create legal discovery and write motions as well as assemble a team of experts and other witnesses, plus prepare direct and cross-examination questions for those who could plead for Will's life. I also received word from the New Jersey Public Defender's Office.

"Mrs. Feldman," began Douglas Smith, head of the office, on a phone call at the end of court that Wednesday, "based on your total lack of experience I will be in court Monday morning to relieve you of your attorney's license due to the attorney prohibition against over-reaching. You have no right to be standing in court on a death penalty case, for God's sake!"

"Mr. Smith, I am caught between a rock and a hard place here. Judge Keichen is demanding that the penalty phase begin on time Monday and my co-counsel has departed for parts unknown. What the hell am I supposed to do?"

"Mrs. Feldman, the rules are very clear. You have violated them. Good day."

I went home and sobbed all night to Rick that my brand new law license would be rescinded at the very beginning of my career for following my obligation to my client. "Honey," soothed Rick, "regardless of what happens Monday, you will have met a high obligation by working for your client. I love you, and I support you."

I spent four days sleeping only an hour a night, preparing for the penalty phase due to begin promptly that Monday at 9:00 A.M. I finished writing my opening statement at 7:00 A.M. that morning, quickly showered, and headed off to court dragging my bulging briefcases on a dolly. In the judge's anteroom, after no sleep and worrying about my law license being taken away by the state public defender's office, I broke down and began to sob. It was 8:45 A.M. and the jury was already seated. Douglas Smith was sitting in the front row with a note pad.

"Lynne," cracked the judge with a smile in an attempt to stem my tears and buck me up in the privacy of his antechamber, "I thought you Texas gals were tougher than that." Judge Keichen had done the trick; I stopped crying, sniffed back the tears, and strode into the court in my power suit and three inch heels, ready for combat.

I was faced with the sole responsibility of convincing 12 good souls that my client didn't deserve to suffer state-sanctioned execution. I had needed help preparing for this critical time, and by utilizing Integral Theory, I wrote my opening and closing statements and addressed the jury. My argument was carefully modeled on Wilber's tenet that "either/or" thinking was a hindrance to the resolution of complex queries. For example, the prosecutor argued that if Will were not given the death penalty, he would not have been adequately punished. This was untrue, since the true duality here was either the death penalty or life in prison. What I attempted to do was dissolve the "either death or not adequately punished" polarity into a "both/and" expression. I argued to each juror as I passed them by during my opening statement that their particular perspective on punishment would most probably resolve into approval for life in prison, and that life in prison was about as bad as being sentenced to death.

One woman had initially expressed her ability to agree with a death sentence when the judge asked her perspective on execution prior to the beginning of our trial. But when I made eye contact with her, now two months later, I spoke of a "both/and" solution. I explained how much my client would be punished by spending his entire life in a six-foot by eight-foot cell. I paced out the space in the courtroom to let them experience how terribly small that space would be, and let her take in the extent of Will's punishment without execution.

To the former Marine with a "law and order" code, I explained passionately that the jury's search for justice could be met with a life sentence, and that inflicting a life term on a 29-year-old virile male would provide sufficient punishment for him as well as sufficient protection for the community from him.

There was a sweet retired librarian who was horrified by my client's crime of strangling his 86-year-old neighbor. The prosecution had argued that Will killed her after she baked him some chocolate chip cookies so he could steal $25 to score crack. I argued to the librarian that justice *and* mercy were two sides of our judicial system. This seemed to resonate with her innate softness toward both the victim and the perpetrator. Each juror nodded affirmatively as I walked by and tried to speak from his or her specific worldview.

After the entire case was presented, and I finally got to do both direct and cross-examination, the jury retired to decide Will's fate. Shortly after going into their locked jury room, they returned with a verdict: my client was not sentenced to death, but to 30 years to life. I had won my first case. Mr. Smith came up to offer me a job with the state public defender's office instead of taking my law license away from me. I thanked him kindly and went home to sleep for several days.

After that heady experience I was offered the position of counsel on the "Iceman" capital murder trial of Richard Kuklinski, a reputed professional hit man who hid his victims in the basement freezer of his home. This trial has been made into a movie called "The Iceman," released in 2013. Having just left a traumatic trial, I opted instead to join a matrimonial firm where my friend Renee Kierey was practicing in 1989, while I kept up a busy criminal practice. I found I possessed an ability to communicate with mentally ill defendants as well as outraged divorce clients, which kept me busy practicing law with Renee on a daily basis. My chameleon-like personality permitted me to relate to individuals in the midst of dire distress. My caring nature consoled my clients, while my protective nature forced me to fight for them with all my might in court. I adored the adversarial nature of the justice system and its creative potential. I could lose myself in the drama and intellectual play of a trial and forget about family and its stresses. Most importantly, I could forget about the real stresses playing out at home and within my family.

CHAPTER SIX

Return of My Mother

On April 4, 1990, I received a call from Florida that I had dreaded for so long: my father had died of a heart attack. One-half of my childhood security net was gone. For a year I keened when I saw a daughter of any age with her father. Where was the daddy I loved and needed? I made arrangements for his body to be buried near my home, and flew to Florida to take my grieving mother and her dog back to New Jersey for the small funeral.

After the rites of mourning had been observed and I began to ease my grief, our biggest question was whether my mother would be able to live alone. I knew I would have to make more frequent trips to Florida to oversee her household and to get her help so she would be able to live independently. I begged my aunts to move to Florida to be near her, but they refused, as much as they complained weekly about Queens and the deterioration of the neighborhood.

Losing my beloved dad, the man who softened the blows of my mother's hysterical behavior with his soft sighs and gentle humor, devastated me. He and I were alike in many ways and I had lost him forever. I turned to my background for spiritual support and began to attend Sabbath services to say the mourner's *kaddish* on his behalf in the summer of 1990. Something stirred in me. I recalled my blissful days singing in our temple choir in Dallas and how the sacred Hebrew words sounded like magic incantations vibrating down to my cells.

I also found solace when I joined our New Jersey temple's choir. Singing the traditional melodies at the High Holy Days lifted my somber spirits into alignment with the transcendent nature of the music. I grew curious about whether Judaism had a unique form of meditation, and discovered there was indeed Jewish meditation and spirituality. I had already begun meditation lessons with Deepak Chopra's lead teacher in 1988, so the strategy of quieting the mind was not new to me. I was given a seed mantra in the Hindu tradition in 1990. Its purpose was to assist me in reaching a transcendent state. By repeating it until my mind fell quieter than normal, I could dive into peaceful minutes. In addition to learning about Jewish spirituality, I investigated other meditation practices for years after my father's death. Some of the practices were conducted in Japanese, others in Thai, Tibetan, Hindi, or Latin tongues. The period after 1990 was a fertile time of investigating different cultures' means of reaching the Divine. I studied each new practice diligently. I was desperate to find a *bhakti* (devotional) path to whichever spiritual lineage I ultimately chose to adopt so I could surrender to the mystery of the Divine.

But I was ultimately frustrated with paths foreign to my background. I then turned to Reb Zalman Schachter-Shalomi's Jewish Renewal (ALEPH) movement. I attended their teachings beginning in 1991, along with their seminars and retreats, and embraced their prayer books and songs. I was now praying in Hebrew, the ancient tongue I heard as a child in temple and transferred through to adulthood in entire services and chantings. I began assisting an Orthodox Rabbi as he wrote a book on Kabbalah in 1992, which deepened my reading, praying, and observing. This rabbi violated his cultural mandate by teaching me, a woman, the most precious form of Jewish mysticism. I was being drawn deeper and deeper into a *bhakti* version of Jewish spiritual practice.

Jewish Renewal endeavored to bring back Judaism's Kabbalistic, Hasidic, musical, and meditative practices. I soon discovered that Reb Zalman was a close friend of Wilber's. Could any practice be better designed for me to deal with my stress and grief? By 1992 I was practicing meditation on a daily basis and absorbing as much as I could from my Jewish roots and community. When my mother came to visit, she, too, embraced spirituality more strongly in the form of nature mysticism. One poem Mom authored that year, entitled "Alpha Visited," is worth quoting:

104

Away from the stones in my breast
And the jagged questions
Escaping through the screwed
Bones and flesh
That hold my cross together
I seek to float out
Beyond the haunches
Where my problems sit,
And join the sky
High, high in soft
Apparitional contentment.
To join the outer rim at some point, pristine
And primitive, far away
From eternal darkness
That breaks world hearts
With weight and misunderstandings;
To rise all in power
Without the dragging body
And the tight cords of reason;
To be threaded to the special tree
With green silk soft as blossoms
Wrapped in nothing brittle
Nor nailed; to be an experience....

We shared books and traded philosophical understandings of Torah and quantum physics into which we had immersed ourselves. I tried explaining Integral Theory to her, but she was a fan of Amit Goswami's theory of the universe as entangled between quantum physics and Eastern mysticism. From a generational perspective, my mother and I were carrying on a tradition begun by her father when he refused to be ordained, yet clung to his roots by arguing Torah with the seminary students.

I was learning Jewish meditation at the time, but felt I "failed" every time I sat down to quiet my mind. This busy-ness of mental chatter is what Buddhists call "monkey-mind." Spiritual practice was important to me, but I kept assuming I was not good enough to sustain any practice. Instead of examining and observing this phenomenon as anchored in severe stress, I merely chalked it up to my inability to meditate. It took years before I could settle into a daily hour session. With my mother somewhat under control, with a burgeoning law practice, and with my daughter's bat mitzvah looming in a few months, I felt relatively happy and challenged.

I even figured out a way to sneak Integral Theory into my childrearing practices. In the 1990s, evangelical Christians took to wearing bracelets with "WWJD?" engraved in the plastic, which stood for "What Would Jesus Do?" I adopted the technique by teaching Erica "WWKWD?" for "What Would Ken Wilber Do?" Not to equate Wilber with a sacred figure, but I wanted to give Erica the rudiments of multi-perspectival awareness. When I asked her "WWKWD?", I was prompting her to look at the situation or question that was perplexing her from three different perspectives: hers, the other person's subjective perspective, and the objective external reality as it occurred to her level of consciousness:

"Mom, Kathy said something nasty to me today about my poem for English. Mrs. McDonald posted all of them on the board."

"What did she say to you?"

"I had a line that read 'when friendships go awry' and she said I misspelled 'away'. I told her she was wrong, I meant what I wrote, and she called me stupid. I felt rotten afterwards."

"Ok, WWKWD?"

"Let's see….First-person point of view is how I felt….I was angry that she criticized my poem at all. Poetry is my personal expression and I'm entitled to say what I think is beautiful."

"Good. You're right on the mark. Now let's think about Kathy's perspective."

"She's entitled to her opinion of what's beautiful too, right?"

"You bet."

"But why does she have the right to make me feel stupid when I used the word correctly?"

"How do you think she was feeling when she made that comment?"

"Hmmm…I think I wrote a really good poem. Maybe she felt jealous and then got happy when she thought I got something wrong."

"Sounds like a good take on the situation. How did you react to

Kathy and her comment?"

"I got hurt right away and left the room. So who won that fight?"

"Do you feel that sort of exchange needs a winner and loser? Is there some other way you could have handled it?"

"I got the word right, but she doesn't know that. So I could have just said that I didn't misspell the word, and walk away."

"What a great way of reframing that, Erica! Good going."

At least in a corner of my life I believed I had reached a plateau of stability and might even make strides in reframing my own convoluted life.

⁕ ⁕

When I unexpectedly received a letter from Central Valley rehiring me in early July 1992, Rick and I first laughed at the idea of leaving my lucrative law practice for teaching. But by the spring of 1992 my mother had come to live with us. She could no longer function alone in Florida even with a home health aide. Except for periods of irrational outbursts over Rick's failure to love my mother or some battle with her sisters, my mother was somewhat quieter after my father died.

Two months after relocating with us, Mom had another psychotic break and was hospitalized at the Bridgewood Hospital psychiatric wing. Unfortunately, that first day she was overmedicated, got up in the middle of the night, stumbled in the room and fell, breaking her hip. She caused daily uproars after being placed in the rehabilitation center by issuing endless complaints about her treatment, the food, her roommate, and the amount of moonlight being admitted into her room through the curtains. A greatly relieved staff permitted her to come to my home for the rest of her recovery.

I had an emotionally challenged person under my roof along with a young child and a husband working two jobs. My mother began to see a psychiatrist in New Jersey who diagnosed her as borderline personality with psychotic episodes plus multiple character and personality disorders and depression. She fit into every category of mental illness. The absence of Melissa did not offer me complete relief; all it meant for me was the replacement of one mentally ill person with another.

We sold my parents' home in Florida and made the proceeds available to my mother. Later, we converted our den and the fourth bedroom downstairs into a suite where she and her dog, Lili, could live in comfort and relative privacy. Things were rocky but I figured having my mother with me might moderate her needs.

The next week I was before a judge in southern New Jersey defending a criminal client when the judge's secretary came running over and handed me a note to call my mother immediately. Alarmed, I excused myself and went into her office to call.

"She sounded desperately ill," cautioned the secretary. "You may need to go right home."

Sure enough my mother could hardly speak. Her voice had no volume and was raspy. "C-c-c-ome right away," she whispered before the phone went dead. I could have called 911 but there was no one home to answer the door and I didn't think she could climb the stairs to answer the first responders. I had my criminal client returned to his cell and sped homeward. I rushed into the house expecting to see a comatose or dead mother on her bed. Instead, she was sitting up with her glasses on and reading the paper.

"Oh, hi there!" she chirped. "I was really getting bored here all alone and I wanted you home. So how did your case go today?"

I was still unable to vent my full outrage at her behavior, and, like my father before me, repressed my fury by stomping back up the stairs to my bedroom, where I flung my briefcase on the floor and called my husband.

"I'm leaving my practice," I hissed into the phone. "I'm going back to teaching. I can't take this any longer!"

"But it'll mean a cut of over half your take-home pay, hon. How will we keep the household going?"

"I can't do this. I'll wind up with an ethics complaint or malpractice charge the way she's interfering with me."

I had made up my mind, and by mid-July 1992, I made the contractual change back to teaching, which would give me shorter hours and two months during the summer to tend to my mother and daughter. My law career thereafter was limited to summers and vacations.

As I have indicated earlier, it was during my years in law school that I became familiar with, and then deeply immersed in, Integral Theory. No one I knew had heard of Wilber at this early point, and I often spent hours at my local Barnes & Noble hoping to meet another person perusing Wilber's books. My plan was to begin a conversation with the other person and maybe have a friend with a similar interest. I was never successful.

It was early September 1992 when I returned to Central Valley High. I decorated my narrow cinderblock-lined classroom with pictures of U.S. presidents and copies of the Constitution. The next day, 26 high school seniors entered the room, drifting in from the humid corridors. Now I had an audience of students. I was free to try out the integral educational theories I was developing. The students were immediately captivated by an integrated presentation of their fragmented course offerings, and implored me to teach them more. The fall months unfolded happily for me at work as I co-created what I envisioned a healthy, integral educational environment would be. I lived for work from 1992 onward, and stayed as late as I possibly could to avoid the havoc at home. I also created exciting new extracurricular activities that took me away from home over long weekends to attend simulated sessions of the United Nations, and hours after school with mock trials. But the situation at home remained fragile, and at any time my routine could be disrupted.

One day in late November 1993, my classroom phone rang. When I picked it up, every student glanced up to see who was about to be called to the principal's office. But it was for me, and I was told to leave my class as soon as a covering teacher arrived, since the police were on the phone.

I raced to the office, afraid that my mother had fallen down the stairs and was injured or dead. Instead, the police informed me that she had notified the cleaning woman she was going to put her head in my oven and kill herself. My oven was electric, so I breathed a sigh of relief upon hearing what the emergency was. Nevertheless, I had to go home and straighten things out with the police who were sitting with my mother in her bedroom.

She told me she was lonely while I was at work, and both Erica and Rick were staying out very late to avoid her. She had a point, so I

109

hired a companion, Maureen, to answer her needs and cook for her while Rick and I were at work.

"Today you are to polish the silver," I heard her command Maureen one day in January 1994. I raced downstairs to warn mom that Maureen was her companion, not the domestic help. Mom didn't seem to care what Maureen's title was; she finally had someone at her beck and call.

Maureen quit a week later after confiding in me, "My doctor told me I am close to having a stroke from your mother and if I intend to live, I'd best get out of your house. I'm so sorry for you and your husband."

A few months later Rick came home while I was at work. Within minutes he was on the phone with me at school and sounding colder than I had ever heard.

"I'm moving out. I am just giving you notice."

"What in God's name happened? We were doing fine at breakfast. What the hell happened?" I shouted back, completely unnerved.

"It's not you, it's your mother! When I came home she was waiting for me in the living room, hands clenched, teeth bared, and face in a death grimace. Then she began to scream at me: 'Where…is…my…money?'"

Rick was too shocked to initially figure out what she was demanding, but the blood drained from his face to hear the viciousness in her voice. He imitated her scary outburst and I was all too familiar with the animalistic tone it took. 'WHERE IS MY MONEY?!? WHERE IS MY MONEY?!?' She repeated it like the battle cry of the undead."

He raced out of our house and called me in a state of utter terror.

"I am not going into that house again with her there. I thought her head was going to spin around and pea soup shoot out of her mouth. Jesus, her money's been in the bank. Where did she think it was?"

"I'd better call 211 before I go into the house."

That service number calls out a psychiatric nurse and trained police personnel to see if the person in question is a danger to himself or others.

110

"What the hell did you do that for?" she screamed when I entered the house and told her what I had done.

"Mom, I have been taking care of your money. I'm a lawyer. I'm your daughter. Nothing has happened to it."

"I don't trust that husband of yours at all. I want proof!"

"That's not a problem, but your behavior is. Neither one of us wants to come back into our own home, mom, and Erica is due home soon. This cannot happen again. We'll get someone to speak with you, and then you and I have to talk."

The mental health squad came. After speaking to her, the nurse addressed me.

"You'd better get help for her immediately. She's mentally unstable but doesn't fit the requirements of a mandatory 72-hour hold in a mental hospital."

Neither Rick nor I wanted to go back to living with my mother. For the first time, I put my foot down when I spoke to her after the nurse left.

"Mom, we'll rent an apartment for you nearby and I will take care of you every day. We'll decorate it just the way you want, but you can't live here any longer."

After much arguing, she agreed to move in the spring of 1995. I spent a great deal of her house proceeds on luxurious appointments for her lovely one-bedroom apartment, which began to resemble our house in Dallas. She secured a rescue cat who kept her company and I found a loving Brazilian woman to be her companion several days a week. I was stressed by the daily and sometimes midnight visits I made to the apartment to deal with her psychological or physical needs, but the peace in our own house was well worth the trouble. That lasted until she had another breakdown.

One summer day the following year in 1996, I called to her upon opening her door and climbed the flight of interior steps to her living room, but only heard grunts. Alarmed, my eyes swept the floor where I encountered her nude body writhing back and forth.

"Mom! For God's sake, what's wrong? Should I call an ambulance?"

"I want to die…I want to die…I want to die..." was all I could get from her.

She was beyond any succor I might offer her, and adhering to emergency protocols, I called 911. She was taken out of her apartment by the police, put in an ambulance, and taken to a local mental hospital. They dismissed her after she created so much turmoil they could no longer contain this 86-year-old woman.

Upon her release she alternated between articulating grateful love for my tender care and ministering to her every need with angry accusations of poor treatment, again with clenched fists and bared teeth.

A week later I entered her house for my daily visit and heard her talking to women whose voices I did not recognize. As I began my climb, I heard her raging and mean voice in mid-sentence: "And she beats me, you know. I am so scared of her. Oh, please help me! I'm just an old woman!"

By the time I had reached the top landing I had three pairs of accusatory eyes focused on me, and a strange woman going "There, there" with her arms around my mother who was noisily sobbing, and shrinking away from me as she saw me.

"What's going on here?" I asked with a catch in my throat. As a lawyer I knew very well where this scene might end.

"I'm Savannah Reynolds, your mother's senior advocate. She's been telling us some very disturbing things about how she is being treated here."

Trying to divert attention away from myself, I offered, "You mean how her landlord wants to evict her because of how she verbally abuses him? I'm the lawyer handling the case and I believe that he will permit her to stay on for another lease renewal."

The other two women shifted in their seats on the golden brocade sofa. It was not a happy-sounding shift, but rather a "harrumph we don't believe you" sound.

"No," responded Savannah with a curt chill in her tone, "I am talking about how you have been physically abusing your elderly mother and how in fear of you she is."

"May I speak to you in private?" I beckoned her with my head toward the kitchen nook with a pleading voice. This was a very serious situation confronting me and I thought if I gave her my mother's psychiatric background I would be off the hook.

112

"No, we will not talk out of your mother's presence. She's the one whose safety we care about." Savannah was not buying anything I was trying to telegraph.

"Look, what if you get permission from my mother to speak to her psychiatrist, Dr. Campbell? Would that help? Then you can do whatever you see fit."

Savannah turned to my mother. "Leah, does that sound fair? Do you feel safe enough to remain here until we speak to your doctor?"

"Oh, please help me," she whimpered, "I'm so scared of her! Just make her go away until later."

Savannah stood in full command of the room. "Lynne, your mother says she is scared of you. Please go away and we will speak to her doctor before we recommend any further action in this case."

I fled, pulling out my cell phone as I descended the steps to the outside door. Upon exiting I called my lawyer friend Janet Lurie.

"Janet?" I shouted, "I may be arrested for elder abuse by this evening. Get ready to act if I call you. I'll tell Rick to be ready with bail, but you have to be ready to get me out promptly and handle this case with the authorities." Janet knew my entire "mother saga" and I didn't have to explain what had occurred.

I was not arrested. The authorities spoke to her psychiatrist, who applauded my efforts in handling a difficult woman. But he told my mother she needed in-patient psychiatric care after what she had just done.

Leah was then off to a Christian hospital where she left a similar wake of chaos. I was called and told to claim my mother, who was being given short notice to find another facility.

"What has she done that you're giving me 24 hours notice?" I asked amidst tears.

Coldly, the hospital administrator informed me,

We tried to give her a new anti-psychotic drug but she threatened the staff. She told them that she was calling you, that you are a lawyer, and that you would have the doctor arrested for senior abuse. I don't care where you take her; just get her out of this facility!

I begged her psychiatrist to take her back to our local hospital ward; he agreed, but the staff would only permit her to stay for a week during which time they would administer five rounds of shock treatment.

Something permanent had to be done. By the grace of God, we found a bed for her at the new and wonderful Jewish Home for the Aged in 1997 where she unhappily, noisily, and slowly slipped away and died peacefully of heart failure in 2002. Aunt Reba had passed away in 1998 and Aunt Debbie passed away quietly in her bed, just as she had wished, in 2005.

I was not present with any of them when they died, and I regret that deeply. Nobel Laureate Joseph Brodsky echoed my feelings when he noted:

> I am saying this not so much out of a sense of guilt as because of the rather egotistical desire of a child to follow his parents through all the stages of their life; for every child, one way or another, repeats his parents' progress. I could argue that, after all, one wants to learn from one's parents about one's own future, one's own aging; one wants to learn from them also the ultimate lesson: how to die. (Brodsky, 1986)

CHAPTER SEVEN

School's Out

I was attending a holiday party at my high school on December 23, 1998, when Rick called me on my cell phone.

"You won't believe this, hon." He rushed his words so quickly that they slurred together. "I was at Dr. Co's for a check-up and he found an aortic aneurysm close to bursting. I need surgery within three months or I'll die." He panted as he continued to explain the doctor's surprising finding.

"You know the heart murmur and the faulty valve that caused me to get SBE [sub-acute bacterial endocarditis] back in 1979?"

"You think I forgot about you spending an entire month in a hospital?" I replied partially out of pique and mostly from worry for this latest health crisis.

"Now the doctor tells me I must have an aortic valve replacement, but he found this aneurysm is so close to the main arteries to my brain that I'm facing something really serious. Shit."

"Shit!" I yelled back at him on the phone, only to have my fellow teachers, who were all in festive moods, yell at me to shut up and get off the phone.

The finest surgeon who specialized in this dual procedure, indeed, the doctor who invented the procedure, was at Mt. Sinai in New York City. We contacted Dr. Griep who agreed to perform the surgery, and Rick underwent seven hours of delicate work on his heart in March 1999.

The operation was a success. Rick eventually made a complete recovery to the point that he won the right to fly again, and immediately joined the Coast Guard Aviation Auxiliary in late 2000. He was responsible for patrolling Manhattan and Long Island Sound in his own plane, which was under the auspices of the Department of Homeland Security. He was not scheduled to patrol on September 11, 2001, but was sent aloft by the government to survey and take pictures of the burning wreckage of lower Manhattan on September 12th. The military needed small planes that could fly low and slow over the twin towers and take reconnaissance-quality photos of what was left. He told me he would be forever scarred by what he saw.

The attacks on the World Trade Center hit me hard emotionally, as they did everyone who lived in our area. Several of my students lost relatives. My neighbors lost their son, Jeremy Glick, when he heroically caused one of the hijacked planes to dive into the ground in Pennsylvania rather than collide with the Capitol or the White House. Jeremy's youngest sister, Joanna, had just transferred to my school. She and I came up with the idea of a civic project called Teen Freedom Corps that would rally students across the nation to be positive role models for their schools, states, and the nation. Within four months we had chapters in eleven states and had appeared on national media to publicize this new venture. We were in touch with the White House's West Wing and its occupants. My aim for the new group was for students to overlook the propensity of "us vs. them" and to consider all of the teens of the world their brothers and sisters. I wanted them to reach out to "others" in a variety of projects keyed to the interest and developmental level of high school students. This is one way in which I wove integral educational theory into my students' lives, and they responded positively to the call.

My subjective reaction to 9/11 was to rethink my spiritual orientation. I began to study Buddhism seriously. My personal library blossomed with shelves of Buddhist classics, and I settled on Zen as my primary orientation. Being an integral practitioner, there was no reason to dispense with my Jewish beliefs or culture; I merely added them to my broadening understanding that all sentient beings had the right to be liberated, happy, and free from pain. After 9/11 I found it difficult to deal with the "us-versus-them" ideation emerging between the Jewish and Muslim communities over who was responsible for the attack. At the dawn of the new millennium, integral spirituality seemed to contain more Buddhist elements than

116

other religions. Being part of a *sangha* and studying the heart sutra made a seamless progression into the integral community. Within both the Jewish and Zen practices I was able to enter into an altered state of "union with all creation," as I had been able to master during my college years.

※ ～

In 2002, two things of seminal importance to my life occurred: my mother passed away of heart failure in her nursing home, and I finally connected with a group of integral practitioners in Boulder, Colorado. Her death hit me quite differently than my father's. I had grieved over her for so many years, had cried tears for hours over her actions or lack of appropriate responses to me, that I felt numb at her passing. I couldn't shed a tear, whereas I cried for hours after my father's funeral. The same week she passed away I finally connected with the integral community, which seemed in hindsight to represent an integrated response to her death and my own rebirth.

Meeting with this group changed my life and brought me the happiest years I had known. Within a few months I was able to meet Ken Wilber in person, and by 2003 I had been asked to join his new Integral Institute. I spent three blissful years riding the whirlwind with an incredible group of people. I created the Center for Integral Education, which at one time had over 300 subscribers to our discussion forum. I still had a full-time teaching job and a part-time legal practice, but I would have given them both up for full-time with the Integral Institute crowd. I was asked to help usher in Integral University as Vice-Chancellor, and was able to meet with an internationally distinguished group of integral scholars. I met some of the finest souls I have ever encountered, and felt I had finally found my "tribe." We worked virtually, over conference calls, and in meetings in Boulder and Denver for three years before financial difficulties, and my own work situation, ended this dream position.

While working at Integral Institute, I found my approach to teaching my own students deepen and broaden immeasurably from what I was learning. I insisted on synthesizing other content areas for my students. They expressed gratitude in hearing how geometry synced with mysticism, and music with anthropology. I just could not seem to find an endpoint where I could rest, such was my love of synthesis and learning.

Between 2003 and 2006 my studies resulted in a list of significant accomplishments. I was Teacher of the Year, appointed by our governor to serve on his character education committee, honored by the state for my work on a character education program after 9/11, honored by our local PBS channel, and by our state legislature for citizenship education. A congratulatory letter from the White House hangs on my wall along with my other institutional honors for creating the Teen Freedom Corps, winning a Horatio Alger Award, garnering coverage in *Teen People*, ABC News, and local publications. My various student teams always brought back trophies and titles, and there was mutual love within the classroom and with their parents. I also did independent research on the latest brain-mind connections to learning, researched an action-inquiry project on an interdepartmental collaboration, and taught my students metacognitive skills. They and I formed a cohesive learning community in my classroom of which I was quite proud.

Professionally, I was able to distinguish between healthy and unhealthy stress, which is differentiated by calling the unhealthy stress "distress" and the healthy, provocative stress "eustress" (Palmer, p. 13). Distress is the negative and destructive condition that I should have stopped in my life, with my family and with my husband's family as well. Eustress is a positive condition and a prod to growth, in which I reveled as I continued to develop sophisticated professional skills in the classroom such as cooperative teaching.

But beginning in 2006, my life seemed to arc away from the happiness that enveloped me since 2002. My teaching career, once the sole refuge of sanity and bliss in my life, gave way to a bombardment of distress that continued until the end of 2007. Schuyler Roberts, the school's beloved social studies chairman at Central Valley High School, retired in June of 2004. He was a courtly man of English descent who referred to even his rowdiest students as "young historians." The students and faculty adored him, and although he never quite understood that I was using integral educational methodologies on my "young historians," he valued my creativity, the manner

118

in which I involved my students in participatory exercises, and their high scores on standardized tests. I was the teacher kids cut school for, only to have them secretly enter my classroom for my lesson lest they miss whatever "was up with Feldman today."

When Schuyler retired, we social studies teachers hoped that our stellar performance as an academic department would be rewarded with an equally wonderful supervisor. Instead, the superintendent of our one-school district hired a very young and inexperienced successor whom the superintendent, Jack Rojo, nicknamed his "attack dog." The faculty saw why this young fellow had been given this role as they witnessed his harsh and dictatorial manner with the whole faculty. He was a 30-year-old social studies teacher from another state, improbably named Pierson (Piers) Boderie (whom the entire faculty called "Bozo" behind his back). Piers was a good six inches shorter than me, and dressed as if he were a professor, complete with bow tie, sweater vest, and jacket, regardless of the weather. Our old principal had retired as well, and moving up into the vacancy in 2006 was a former (and hostile) colleague of mine from the chemistry department, Richard (Dick) Kaiser.

Central Valley High is a strange creation of New Jersey home rule. It is a one-school regional high school district formed by two towns that have their own elementary schools. The tiny school has its own board of education as well as a full-time superintendent and principal, all within one very modern glass enclosed structure on a rolling bucolic campus surrounded by corporate headquarters. Our students often apprenticed within the corporations, and the C.E.O.s lectured to our business classes.

In true hierarchical form, the superintendent, principal, and department supervisors ruled over the 120 teachers (and 1,400 students) who had little hope of appeal if the three administrators decided to line up against an individual teacher. I saw that scenario play out many times. But as a highly praised senior teacher in the social studies department, I thought I was "safe" from any retribution for speaking honestly and earnestly to this new, inexperienced supervisor on behalf of my peers. At least that was how our school had functioned previously. I had two years left in my teaching career before I could retire with full pension and continue my integral, legal, and spiritual education careers. I felt I would not be harassed as per the fears of my junior colleagues.

I was very wrong. I entered a time at work of such bleakness and woundedness it still inspires nightmares. Jealousy, revenge, power maneuvers, and my own missteps all came into play in a situation where I had no means to fight back or even leave the game.

It began early on during the transition, when various department members felt threatened by Boderie. They asked me to take their grievances to the principal, which I naively did. I encountered Dick in a long sunlit hallway one day and asked for a moment with him.

"Dick, did you know that Anita and Paula were in tears after Piers ripped them apart over little issues with their lesson plans?" I asked as we stood by our department's office entrance. He had a stack of papers under his arm and sweat on his upper lip. His red toupee was a different shade of hair color from what hair he had left. I casually wondered why he didn't match up the colors to better hide the nature of his artifice. "Could you maybe talk to him and tell him how we like to give positive comments as well as negative comments when we get our evals?"

"You aren't the supervisor, Lynne. I have no interest in what you are suggesting. You have no training as a supervisor." He spun on his heels with his chin in the air and left me with my mouth open. I thus earned the ire of both Dick the principal, and Piers my supervisor.

The first direct confrontation with Piers involved his continuing practice of humiliating and deprecating our teachers in public and private. We had the highest scores of any department on the various state and national assessments our students took, and the highest positive rating of any department among students and parents. None of us in the department could understand why we were singled out for this type of demeaning treatment. Even common courtesy was missing from our treatment. This time I went directly to Piers. He was seated in our department office and I took the chair next to him.

"Piers, you know the qualification tests for the advanced placement courses you want us to administer and grade next week?"

"What are you saying to me, Lynne?" he shot back defensively.

"We used to proctor and grade them as a courtesy to Schuyler, and he was so sweet that he gave us coffee and donuts."

"That has nothing to do with me, Lynne." His face was devoid of emotion but I could see the veins on his neck begin to enlarge and turn red.

"But you know we have lunch at 10:30 A.M.; school is out at 3:00 P.M. and we proctor until 6:00 P.M. Then we go home and we return the graded tests by the next day. Remember that we're not being paid for this time and effort. Schuyler brought us refreshments to tide us over, and to thank us. Do you think you might remember to bring us something to nosh?"

He bolted up from his chair and strode over to the door, spun on his heels to glare at me, then turned around and stalked out into the hallway.

After several more "reminders" from me about acting with a modicum of appreciation, Piers did show up with some refreshments for our unpaid labor, but thereafter I became the target of nasty remarks.

I thought I had been respectful in my request, which turned out to be quite a mistake. This was not my job and I should not have inserted myself into others' issues, but this was how all senior department members had behaved since I joined the faculty.

Within two months I found myself moved from my ground floor wall-to-wall glass classroom overlooking hills and groves of trees into the smallest and hottest room in our otherwise bright and airy building. Fresh tar on the ceiling outside my lone small window with no view gave off fumes that caused headaches for both me and my students. My professional assessments changed from exemplary to subpar within a year. The biggest accusation lodged against me was that I was "student-centric."

This did not mean I was performing perfectly. Superintendent Rojo told me he would take his "attack dog" Piers off of me if I filed my intention to retire in 2008; I didn't trust Rojo's word, having heard from others that he reneged on many such arrangements, and so I refused to file my formal notice. That angered him immensely. I also found myself chronically fatigued during the day for lack of sleep at night due to stress (and undiagnosed severe sleep apnea), and I made many grading errors. But whatever my missteps, they did not qualify me for the daily harassment I came to experience beginning in 2006.

I once brought a thermometer into class to register the sweltering June heat, and saw it spike well over 100 degrees. I went to my colleague George.

"Hey, George, your air-conditioned classroom is empty next period, isn't it?" I asked.

"Yup."

"Mind if I hold class in it? I can't even breathe in mine and three kids had to go to the nurse this morning."

"No prob, it's yours. Hot as hell today. Whew," he commented as he mopped his sweat-ridden balding head with his handkerchief.

Within an hour, Piers had accosted me in our department office. With clenched fists and teeth bared, he snarled in a deep animalistic guttural voice as he approached me, "How…dare…you! Only *I* have the power to permit you to switch rooms for one period. You had no right going directly to George!"

"But he said I could, Piers, and Dick told us to get cool however we could manage," I could barely whisper back.

He continued to advance on me with fists thrust toward me and his face contorted and red. His neck veins were distended and gurgling sounds of rage emanated from his throat.

I stepped backwards for a few paces as he advanced, then turned and fled the room in fear for my physical safety. I began shaking uncontrollably and feeling devoid of living warmth, such was my chill. I considered calling the police but felt helpless, and with no other witnesses I figured no one would believe what just happened.

This distress took a toll on my physical and emotional health. I suffered a stroke in my retina after another threat by Piers in the hall in front of my colleagues. This left me out of work for two weeks. Piers called me at home, not to say he felt badly about causing the stroke, but to challenge whether I actually had one at all. "Want to see the pictures the doctor took of the blood clot?" I finally snapped back at him.

But suffering a stroke in my eye did nothing to stem his ongoing abuse.

"I just received a call from Mrs. Strongby that she called you *five times* and you never returned one of them!" he shouted in the hallway during passing period so that both students and my fellow teachers heard and observed. My students scuttled into my class-room like little mice afraid of a lurking cat.

"No, Piers, she called me and I called her right back. We had such a positive exchange that she wants to have coffee with me next week."

"Don't you dare call me a liar!" he screeched. "She called you *five times* and you never called her back!"

"I've got her call still recorded on my phone and the record of when I called her back. Do you want to call her and verify what I just told you?"

"*YOU ARE IMPOSSIBLE!*" he raged, and stormed away down the hall. I had to return to my 12th-grade students and deflect their fear of Piers.

"Who is that man?" Antoinette asked as she peered into the hall after Piers' retreating figure.

"I don't like him. Don't ever let him in your classroom, ok?" said Jason. It was a hard issue for me to navigate with my 7th period. Piers had every right as my supervisor to enter my classroom and "write me up" every day, as he wound up doing.

One "offense" I committed was turning my back on my students when I went over to the board to turn off the light to show a movie on our white board. I purportedly showed "disrespect" by turning my back on them and "failed to keep the class under constant sur-veillance."

I gave half credit to an answer on a "fill in the blank" test when a student answered "Bill of Rights" instead of "First Amendment" when the question read: "What granted us the right of freedom of speech?" Piers confiscated all of my tests before I could hand them back and made me regrade each one of the 120 tests so that *his* ver-sion of the one and only correct answer would be counted. For that I was told I had to attend remedial teaching classes during the fall semester.

On another occasion, Dick called me into his large principal's office at the very back of the building with his degree from a never-heard-of college in a huge frame, and ordered me to sign a statement for my permanent file ordering me to cease teaching creatively.

"Lynne," he stated in his supercilious manner as he leaned over his desk towards me, "this creative teaching must stop. I just want lectures, and from now on you are to provide me with a word-for-word script from which you will teach each class every day, in addition to your lesson plans. I want one-word answer, fill-in-the-blank, and multiple choice question tests, with one simple paragraph for an essay. You give too many points for the students' essay responses. And I never want to see another creative assignment from you again!"

I began getting asthma and bronchitis attacks on a weekly basis. During this period of ill health I was given written chastisements that were put in my permanent record for all manner of alleged misdeeds; my small incremental raise was withheld so that my pension would be smaller; and the superintendent formally informed me that they were going to deprive me of my tenure so they could fire me in my 25th year. Our entire faculty was supportive of me and came to whisper their feelings when the administration was not around. Indeed, when some of the teachers were threatened to write false accusations against me, they flat-out refused.

I could not take the stress any longer, and in the fall of 2007 I hired a top employment discrimination lawyer to fight for me. After substantiating what I had been living through, he told me my situation was the worst case of workplace harassment he had seen in his long career against major corporations. The mistreatment escalated, with new charges against me being lodged every day.

After my weekly trip to my general practitioner, Dr. Bennett took me by the shoulders and said gravely, "Lynne, this stress has shut down your immune system. Do you really understand the severity of your health situation?"

"But I have to stay on the job until this situation is settled. If I leave now, I won't get my full pension or lifetime healthcare." I had no energy to continue this legal fight, but there didn't seem to be any way out of it.

"Then settle *now*, Lynne, this very month, or you won't live to retire in June!"

I couldn't believe what my doctor was telling me about not living another six months under the stress I was experiencing. This was my ultimate nightmare: dying on the job due to abuse, humiliation, and scapegoating.

"Lynne, please don't give up this case," begged the paralegal John. "We are looking at a heavy six-figure verdict we're pretty confident you'll win. Can you just hang in there for a few more months while we get ready for trial?"

"No, I really can't," I informed John and the rest of my top-notch legal team. "We'll have to settle the suit or else I won't survive. I have no wiggle room here for legal maneuvering." They tried their best to get me to fight onward, but the doctor's words were harsh and absolute: settle or die.

We did settle. I left teaching on December 21, 2007, after our initial hearing in court, where I was sick physically and emotionally. It took a few more weeks to finish up the legal matters during which I never set foot in my classroom at Central Valley. Indeed, I never set foot in the school again. After 24 and a half years of devotion to my profession and my students, I was out. But I did not feel relieved of the stress; rather, it was as if my body had collapsed. I was without an identity again and without a reason to be alive.

CHAPTER EIGHT

An Integral Approach

"What do you plan to do now that you're retired?" asked my daughter as we sat around my kitchen table in 2008.

I didn't know, and I certainly didn't feel retired. There was no closure, no retirement party or dinner in my honor, no declaration from the Board of Education with gratitude for my nearly 25 years of service and countless awards.

The best move I made during this time was to get a puppy, Chloe, and let her lavish her unconditional love all over me. Rick and I managed to stitch together our battered marriage once the stress of the school situation was finally over. He became my number one cheerleader and support person throughout the school (and medical) ordeals. I continued my legal career and received certification in special education law and alternative dispute resolution. I traveled to Costa Rica and the Galapagos on my own in 2010 and awaited the beginning of my new spiritual program in New York City. My future seemed to have taken a positive turn, one that might carry me well into my last years of productivity.

But stress continued to rob me of sleep and tranquility. I had continuous nightmares that I was being harassed once again. I dreamed I had nowhere to turn, and no one to stand up for me. In real life at the time, the faculty was so excited I was going up against the administration, until the eyewitnesses realized they'd have to testify on my behalf. They then declined to take the stand after witnessing the harassment I had endured; they were understandably self-protective.

I sat there in the kitchen with my smiling child, now a happily married woman and successful attorney. I couldn't answer her owing to the lump in my throat; my stomach was as tight as a string mop being wrung out. How could I address Erica's query about my future when I was still dealing with the heavy stress wracking my body?

Stress is an invasion of personal integrity, and mine had been invaded since my birth. People and situations put demands on my boundaries as an individual self, and throughout my life I had been asked/coerced to give into those demands and invasions. Unfortunately, how I attempted to deal with those invasions served me less and less well as I matured. Giving into a demanding and mentally ill mother can be understood as a survival mechanism when I was a little girl. Continuing to give into her as a grown, married woman was not a healthy response. Giving into others who invaded my self-sense as an adult was also not a good strategy for my growth or health.

Once I had been diagnosed, I thought back over my lifetime of significant stresses that I began to see as the probably provocateur of my cells that mutated into cancerous lesions in parts of my body. Two years after I left teaching, I could have chosen a lifetime of episodes as the most stressful. I could also lump them together as a *chronic series of acute stresses*. Any one of them made me expend tremendous energy to push back. I believe this energy depletion deprived my immune system of the capacity to maintain a safe boundary between me and the world outside of me.

"Mom, why are your hands shaking?" Erica asked as I tried to stir my milk into my coffee that day, with the contents sloshing over the lip.

I wasn't sure why my hands had began shaking, so off to a neurologist I went in the winter of 2008.

"Have you been under any stress lately?" asked Dr. Molina in a professional tone. I responded with almost manic laughter. It startled her, and she asked me to recount what I had been through recently. After narrating my situation with the school, she concluded my shaky hand signified, in layman's terms, that I was a nervous wreck. She suggested I do something fun to rejuvenate my psyche and return me to the realm of satisfied living.

Following doctor's orders, I booked a wonderful trip to Spain with my school friends in March 2008. But I had to cancel when the week before departure I was diagnosed with pneumonia that left me in the hospital for respiratory treatment.

Although I could acknowledge that I was indeed a "nervous wreck," the boundaries between me and reality never broke. In other words, I never had a nervous or psychiatric breakdown, nor had I been diagnosed with anything more severe than generalized anxiety. My other bodily systems were strained to fracturing, however, which made me vulnerable to a continuous series of bronchial infections. I believe these physical and emotional strains caused my immune system to be compromised and rendered it unable to recognize and eradicate mutating cells.

"The research indicates that stress—maybe even the stress of being cold—appears to tap into the same immune system-nervous system loop that triggers symptoms of the common cold," according to Steven Maier, Ph.D. Maier considers stress to be another form of infection, a specifically severe form, since it can short-circuit the very mechanisms our bodies have developed to filter out infections from our cells. In fact, depressed mood produces all the same behavior changes as both the sickness and stress responses.

It was two years after my battle with the school that I got my diagnosis of breast cancer. As much as I might have liked to find a *direct* link between my unending life stress and my diagnosis of breast cancer, there is none. Dr. David Servan-Schreiber, in his excellent book *Anti Cancer: A New Way of Life* reminds us as recently as the 1980s any mind-body connection was ridiculed by the medical establishment (2009, p. 146). Today, medical practitioners are far more likely to admit such a connection, but to say that life stress is the only cause of cancer would be *quadrant absolutism*, in integral parlance, which means believing that only the subjective-interior "I" operates on our body/minds. Dr. Servan-Schreiber is adamant when he asserts:

> I must insist on one point: No psychological factor
> *by itself* [emphasis added] has ever been identified

as being capable of creating that bad seed. In other words, nothing permits us to state that psychic trauma can be the sole cause of cancer.

Yet, as with nutrition, exercise, or the quality of our air and water, he states equally emphatically that certain psychological states can indeed profoundly influence our immune systems. I might have had a genetic propensity for these cancers, but I believe life and workplace stress accelerated the mutations. Did pointing to stress as the causative factor of the cancers give me a sense of having more control over my destiny? Was I following in my mother's path when she was sure she could spot the person who gave her bronchitis? Was I adding more "should haves" to my life?

If anything, I "should have" devoted more attention to caring for myself. But my mother and her family attacked me when I tried to do just that, and called me out for my "selfish behavior". I was continually reminded that my reason for being alive was to be in service to my mother and her family. Considering my repressed upbringing, the malevolent treatment by my mother-in-law, the extenuating circumstances involving raising Melissa, and my stress on the job, I existed in a chronic state of acute stress. In Parker Palmer's words, "There are times when the heart, like the canary in the coal mine, breathes in the world's toxicity and begins to die" (2011, p. 3). How could I continue to deal with the toxicity in my life if I did not pay attention to my body and my heart?

The word "heart" stems from its Latin root "cor," which suggests it is my heart that is the very core of my self. The core integrates my meaning-making ability and my sense of the world—my intuitive, imaginative, emotional, relational, spiritual, physical, and intellectual ways of knowing (Palmer, p. 6). And "cor" is also the root for "courage." I entered the realm of cancer at low personal ebb. My heart felt mortally wounded. Unbeknownst to me, so were my cells. By 2010 I would have to integrate all my abilities, and show courage as I had never known before.

There was one curative method available to me, but I wasn't at a physical or psychological state to apply it yet: the way through the trauma of stress, helplessness, and a sense of victimhood is *to harness the passion of grief.* It was not by adopting the guise of hardy Lynne who was known to heroically brave all of my life's vicissitudes for decades. Early on, I had learned to don a smiley face regardless of what chaos and pain seared inside. Rare was the compassionate soul who really wanted to hear of my troubles; some even called me to cheer themselves after hearing of my latest trauma. This guise of the happy warrior did not help me rally energy to fight my mortal illness. I had to learn to lean into my pain, to grieve my abnormal and unhealthy upbringing, and the loss of a stable professional and personal life. By letting my aching sense of loss experience the pain that was submerged within me, I felt more spacious awareness by which to aggregate energy for this fight.

Were it not for the onset of cancer, I might have comfortably spent my retirement beginning in 2008 sorting through my personal conundrums and settling down to a life well examined. But in truth I was barely functioning. As for emotional and therapeutic interventions, I am not naturally a depressed person. But this extraordinary level of stress led me to doubt my value in the world. I would not have taken my own life, but if something had come along (as it did), I might not have fought against it.

Looking for somatic work, I quite accidentally found Lorraine Antine in 2009, who practiced holistic energy psychotherapy. She described her work in this manner:

> Holistic Energy psychotherapy is based upon the theory that traumatic memories and the negative beliefs, emotions, and behaviors that often result from them are experienced as energy blocks in the human energy field. By introducing techniques and tools into therapy that help to restore balance to our energy field, many psychological and emotional problems often resolve rapidly and fully, never to return! ... In many respects, the sessions are very similar [to traditional psychotherapy].... The difference resides primarily in the choice of interventions used during the course of treatment and the focus on wellness, rather than pathology. (Holistic Integrative Therapies, 2014)

I did not initially understand what she provided, but she did understand I had lived a life of trauma, generalized anxiety, and we began to work together in depth psychology along with her intuitive healing. As it turned out, she was one of those practitioners who may not have studied integral theory but who practiced it and embodied it nonetheless.

Lorraine and I dug deeply into what she saw was the origin of my victim mentality; my family and marital history were unearthed in all of their raw pain that I often thought of quitting. Why continue in a therapy that causes as much pain as I felt going into it, I wondered? But ferreting out areas of emotional pain became a critical part of my healing journey. Like lancing and cleaning an infected area of the body, I was able to begin emotional health and energy.

Creating a program at a local seminary kept me busy and feeling less depressed. But this was a pseudo-solution to my emotional state, I later discovered. My coping mechanism has always been to get busy to avoid feeling depressed or smothered. This activity heightens my adrenaline rush and gives me the illusion that I am feeling buoyant and "myself again." Not knowing what else to do, I immersed myself in creating a new way of being in spiritual service by using Integral Spirituality. I made plans for 2008 through 2010(which would be interrupted by my cancer diagnoses)to become an interfaith minister. These plans blew up in my face when I tried and failed to maintain the schedule and pace of creating and teaching a new program. From 2010 through 2012, I was in a state of denial about how weak and compromised my body and psyche actually were. I may have thought I had passed through the *lightning strikes*, but I was nowhere near *coming to terms* with my situation.

I kept busy and committed to this new program, and was trying in vain to put psychic distance between my wounded will and me. I was also trying to deal with the accumulation of wounds from my family of origin, my in-laws, and outsiders which almost crippled me psychologically. I was born with a desire to please, to do what I had promised. Yet something didn't feel right to me while working with such effort on my program while feeling so ill. I had a sneaking suspicion that I was mere replacing one source of stress with a new source. Somewhere inside, I considered I should have permitted myself to heal in quiet from this latest assault rather than launching into yet another trying situation, which ultimately handed me a mountain of problems.

This was a return to the busy-ness coping strategy I had always employed and how I repressed my life's sorrows. I wanted to be happy and retain my generativity by creating new programs as I had done in my legal and teaching careers. And thus I drove myself right back into a lack of rest and renewal.

But then cancer forced me into an entirely new phase of my life. In 2010, cancer upended all of my carefully crafted post-teaching events, and reawakened the dreaded idea that perhaps my life was indeed cursed by bad fortune. Cancer forced me into an ongoing radical self-honesty as I was repeatedly rocked by frightening news of my health. Rather than relaxing into my sixties as a spiritual educator, I had to recalibrate who and where I was: I was living on the edge, between life and death, and had to figure out how to live with wildness. I realized this wildness could propel me, at last, to find and anchor myself to my unique self. The shocks of the *lightning strikes*, which increased every month from diagnosis for almost two years, both debilitated and awakened me to that which was at my core.

How was I going to approach my new situation psychologically and cognitively? Was this another phase of the Greenberg curse? Did I have a core spiritual belief system that might support me? I did indeed have such a core: integral spirituality. My beliefs were part of my *first-person subjective* perspective and formed my thoughts whenever I said things like "I believe that the Divine…" Yet I found myself wishing I believed in an all-powerful Diety "up there" somewhere, who would talk to me and help me decide how to approach my treatment. I felt jealous of those folks who could trust such messages from an all-knowing, paternal figure.

I needed to burrow as deeply as I could into what I held unconsciously as well as consciously about my place in the universe. If I had whole-heartedly accepted that I was one with the One, then that belief system would support me in a search for a healing program. But I felt fingers of cold doubt separating what I thought I believed from what I feared as they tussled for dominance.

My other option would be to decide that the universe had no value whatsoever, no intention, no meaning, no depth, and no quality, and thus I might isolate my choices to the physical realm of medical treatment alone. Most of what I read about breast cancer treatments pushed the patient to "scientize" her experience into a *third-person objective* perspective: "It is the truth that surgery..." What would happen to me if I agreed that science alone and above all domains could suffice to lead me through my healing journey? This embrace of "scientism" is prevalent in both of my fields of expertise, teaching and law. After all, who can argue with an x-ray, blood test, DNA evidence or image of the brain? If I chose this perspective on healing, what role would be left to me in my choice of treatment regimen?

I read that a total mastectomy gave me the best odds for surviving the cancer that resided within me. But I intuitively felt there were other factors that might increase my chance of survival, such as nutrition, exercise, massage, support groups, and meditation. Instead of an "either/or" approach of surgery versus other modalities, I decided I would do both to the fullest extent possible: use holistic therapies as well as undergo the right physical treatment to rid my body of cancer.

This embraced a "both/and" approach, but did not mean I had to choose surgery if I didn't want it. I could have opted for a complementary or alternative healing approach, but it would require I would have to abide by whatever protocols or practices those treatments held as true. I also had the option of adding alternative methods to the establishment protocols and practices, but I would have to be cautious that one method did not cancel out or exacerbate the other.

I am a professional researcher, trained lawyer and educator. I have practiced in and written for both of these communities, and am familiar with their cultural values. When I step into my local county court house, I know that women may wear a variety of outfits, whereas in southern jurisdictions, suits or dresses are the cultural norm. I therefore abide by a second-person "we" perspective: "We do not wear slacks to court." The cultural "We" factor is often ignored or enters our decision-making unconsciously. But I was aware of the cultural bias in my geographical area in favor of "scientism."

If I wanted to mix and match traditional medical treatments with complementary and alternative methods, I would have to be ready to push the doctors to appreciate my wishes.

I understood that I could marry the "I," "We," and "It" understandings of my moment-to-moment reality about my illness. This would mean I would be looking to the great wisdom traditions' approach to healing, and to the wisdom and the science that existed for deciding what decisions I should make. This would be my integral approach.

I would apply integral theory and create a healing practice that would embrace everything we know to be true and good about fighting my illness—not just one aspect of the solution. Instead of just eating organic foods, or just relying on surgery, or thinking positive thoughts, I would construct an overarching and almost limitless approach to attacking that which was attacking me. Upon registering this affirmative statement, my battle plan had been set forth. I did feel overwhelmed, however, as I realized I would have to do this on my own, by myself.

When integral is practiced as a holistic system, the secret seeds of its deepest implication of Wilber's words and protocols spark together to grow into something beyond normal understanding, and provoke more than normal behavior. I had wanted to return to that state of "psychoactive" bliss that integral practice opened up to me at an integral seminar in 2003. I wanted to reside in that state permanently, or at least dwell in that state for a longer period of time.

If I wanted to embrace all areas of my consciousness and harness them for healing, I could not repress or ignore my darkest recesses or the most injured aspects of my traumatized self. The mutual enrichment of combining science with psychology and spirituality in my healing journey would have to incorporate 100% of the physically supported path as well as 100% of the psychological and spiritual path (i.e., *not* a 50/50 proposition, but 100/100).

I discovered from my research that we are at a fulcrum shift in our approaches to treating cancer patients. We are shifting from the strictly uniform "one size fits all" medical model to a carefully individualized treatment regimen, and more cancer facilities are including alternative and complementary healing modalities.

Other emerging approaches which fascinated me were narrative medicine and writing for healing, which led me to begin my blog and then write this book. These approaches are becoming popular due to complaints from both the medical and patient communities that treatment comes from physicians trained solely in the scientific, objective third person perspective. Our medical issues are dealt with merely as "mechanical/biological" problems to be solved. There is no room in this model for inquiry or concern with the psychological and personal history of the patient. By encouraging both medical practitioners and patients to tell and share their personal stories, a holistic approach to healing opens up between them. This is an ideal time for practitioners and institutions to look into the integral model of medicine, but also for me to create an individualized healing program as I did. Patients should not have to choose between an exclusive reliance on science and reliance on anything other than science.

As I spoke to my friends, and as acquaintances learned about my diagnosis, I was once again confronted with the "either/or" sentiments most people seem to hold. I spoke to one massage therapist who pooh-poohed any of the modern medical approaches I was considering initially.

"Lynne," he advised me as we sat with friends at an organic café over lunch the day after my diagnosis, "why would you permit dangerous surgery and toxic chemicals to enter your body? Don't you know that the chemicals they give you for chemo create further cancers and destroy all of your healthy cells? That's just insane. Listen to your friends…I promise I will massage the tumor away. Just come by my office and forget surgery."

Another friend warned me, "You'd better get rid of those negative thoughts about yourself that you've been uttering. Your positive beliefs and intentions alone can cure you of any type of cancer at any stage, but your negative thoughts can doom you." I saw through the pitfalls of this way of viewing things. I was more interested in achieving a balance of both. *What's wrong with my embracing spiritual practices along with the standard treatments of surgery, radiation, and chemotherapy?* I kept wondering. *And where will I find caregivers who will understand what I am aiming for?*

The experience of facing a disease that might lead to death required me to embrace the counterintuitive understanding that the world is a gift where we co-create and experience its abundance, wholeness, and interdependence. What other choice did I have? Otherwise, I would sit at the white table in my kitchen adorned by 20 of my mother's riotously lush oil paintings of nature, and be grimly despondent. I could embrace this fullness and abundance if I turned to the three seminal categories of "being in the world": acknowledging that there exists a Good, a True, and a Beautiful. Every moment, every breath, every thought reflects my acceptance of these three categories. They are open to my changing what belongs in which category, but I possess all three concepts at all times. Since they are so basic, it is where I began my quest for healing.

The Beautiful is my first-person perspective. "Beauty is in the eye of the beholder" is its motto. I allowed myself to sink into the brushstrokes before me laid down 60 years before, which my mother administered while sitting in her art studio as I looked on, fascinated. I entered into the lushness of her personal representation of flowers and birds, and regardless of the piles of snow by the kitchen door, I was at one with nature. Perhaps a visitor might not like her paintings, but I adored each one and found healing when I stared at them.

Healing could begin by embracing the Beautiful around me at all times, whether it was art, music, or even retail therapy. At this watershed time in my life, I found it to be a critical component. I sang along with Rabbi Shefa Gold's Hebrew chants, and I felt connected to her and to the choir of voices that joined her. I screamed out Billy Joel's music and was then lulled into tranquility by my classical collection. I splurged on clothes that would fit my new body shape after my surgery. At any time of despair or period where the gift of life seemed like a sham, I could repair myself by sinking into that which satisfied my desire for beauty.

The Good emanates from a second-person perspective; it embraces what you and I together believe about our culturally dictated/absorbed values. When I join my family for a spontaneous Chinese dinner or an elaborately planned holiday celebration, I exist within the container of values and culture. I feel enveloped yet never ensnared, and we know our laughter is a joint chorus to life's fullness and pleasure. Nothing felt more healing than my infant grandson's soft breathing as he slept nestled in my arms, and nothing nourished me more than a gathering of my husband, daughter, and son-in-law as we recounted the week's events. We were engaged in relational well-being (i.e., a shared and savored the meaning of what is good for us and our culture).

A trickier aspect of the Good which I had to sort out was to decide it would benefit my family, my community, and me personally to continue to be alive on this earthly plane. My sense of self-worth had been so muted that I had times when I wondered if I would be missed if the cancer took me quickly. I also realized that my frenetic escapism had cost me old and dear friendships. I had neglected them, and now I wanted to repair them. I reached out to them, so many loving people, and they welcomed me back. I saw in their deep concern for me that I was still an important part of a "we" community, and I returned to my former place within it.

Then there was Melissa. I had been seriously traumatized by her mental illness and its attendant conduct disorders. There were many years when we hadn't spoken, as I laid blame for the disunity with my husband's family at her door for having lied about me and Rick. But as I began my spiritual practice, I came to accept that I could no more hold her responsible for her actions while she was so young and ill than I could condemn my mother for hers. Slowly, tentatively, we began reaching out to one another on a different level. In 2008 our daughter Erica married Simon, and Erica reached out to Melissa and her daughter to not only attend her wedding, but for the daughter to be a junior bridesmaid. Thanks to Erica's hand of reconciliation, Melissa and I embraced on the dance floor and commenced our healing after many years. This softness would have to grow as a central part of my personal healing. I could not risk the old hot anger remaining in my heart.

From my objective third-person perspective of what was True, I reached out to science and nature. What is True in our era is empirical—based on peer-reviewed material, double-blind tests, and mathematical and medical findings. I did not doubt the surgeon's diagnosis of my illness since he was applying protocols relied upon by the top cancer hospitals throughout the world. His fellow oncologists agreed with the diagnosis, and when he laid out my treatment plan, I knew and trusted that thousands of doctors and scientists had collaborated upon these very procedures. Hundreds of thousands of patients had undergone the recommended treatments, and I could look up survival statistics based on double-blind studies.

Each of us is aware of the three dimensions in the manifest world: I can see myself as the "I"; my friend Robin and I share an event within a "We space"; and I can talk about things or facts existing as an "It." As I read the studies for breast (and later lung) cancer, trying to make sense of the researchers' arcane terminology and sometimes contradictory findings, I knew that in time I would settle on a scientific truth I could follow.

I was also aware that most of the doctors I would consult, regardless of their brilliance, would privilege the True and generally dismiss the spheres of the Beautiful and the Good as medical healing modalities. On the other hand, some cancer healing providers refuse to acknowledge the vast findings of the "hard" health sciences and choose instead to apply the Good or the Beautiful to their clients' metastasizing cancers. I needed all of them together.

Where might I place the belief system that all who have cancer are "victims"? This fed into my belief I bore some type of mythic/magic, familial bad luck—the "Greenberg curse." Was it part of my personal spiritual beliefs or from larger cultural beliefs? It did not fit into the True way of being in the world; thus, it must be part of my personal and cultural systems.

If it wasn't true, then I could change my belief. My healing plan would become an opportunity for me to transform this limited sense of my self as victim into a transcendent belief of an all-encompassing Self. It would be joined with all the other sentient beings, feel their pain and their joy, and go beyond what is happening in my local body. It could be reached by continuing my spiritual practices, or just by landing upon me like a strike of grace. It would not mean giving up my "self", the individuated "Lynne" living a "Lynne-life" along with the transcendent Self.

I held a means by which to overcome my long-held victim mentality during the course of my treatment. I had to tread one step at a time, and my next step was to enter Sloan-Kettering and meet the man who would be my surgeon. The True, the Good, and the Beautiful would be my guides through this coming phase of my illness.

CHAPTER NINE

Medical Strikes

As I entered Sloan-Kettering in October 2010 to meet my new surgeon, it exceeded my vision of what a world-class research hospital might look like. Each floor was equipped with the Internet, beverages and snacks, and knowledgeable staff. The facility was tastefully decorated with soft oil paintings and lithographs, and had a color scheme reflecting the polarities of hope and despair. I would have been offended by an overly cheery choice of tropical colors if I were receiving a terminal diagnosis, yet too bland a choice would have pulled me down into fretful ruminations of bad news.

Before I entered the elevator, I picked up a pamphlet supplied by the women who ran the Resources for Life After Cancer program. These groups were tailored to give cancer survivors an opportunity to work on personal and practical concerns by taking an active approach to their medical issues. *No way are you near that stage yet*, I cautioned myself, but I picked up a leaflet anyhow. There, in bold letters, was this description of one support group:

Grace & Grit: A Women's Circle: A weekly group providing women cancer survivors an opportunity to share concerns while taking a problem solving approach.

Wilber and integral were alive and well at Sloan-Kettering, perhaps without knowing about Wilber's book of the same name. I pledged myself to make Wilber's work known to them, which I did in the spring of 2003 when I handed the social worker a copy of *Grace and Grit.*

My husband and I met Dr. Sacchini in his well-ordered office. He turned out to be a soft-spoken, gentle, Italian physician who had the sad eyes and speech of a person who has seen more than his share of pain. I found this both oddly endearing and frightening. Would I be one of the patients he would recall with sorrow for my quick passing, or with humility for having cured me?

He looked over my scans and told me, "Your tumor measures 2.3 x 1.3 centimeters, but when I palpated your breast, I could not feel it. This is good, Lynne, it doesn't present as a hard solid mass even though we know it is cancer and we know it has invaded healthy tissue. Let's find out if it has stayed where it is, or if any cells have migrated to the sentinel lymph node."

I had already done a cursory Internet search of terms associated with breast cancer, but I asked him to explain what that meant.

Dr. Sacchini continued, "That's the node under the arm pit which is the first to filter out bacteria and other toxins on their way to the general blood stream. If there is cancer in the sentinel node, then we have to cut out more lymph nodes until we get to a cancer-free zone. But the more nodes with cancer we find, the greater the odds the cancer has had access to your bloodstream and might have already traveled elsewhere."

My first needle biopsy at Heights had reported there was no cancer past the original mass, so I felt comforted that this next test would not reveal further frightening news.

I underwent a new needle biopsy at Sloan-Kettering right away, and Dr. Sacchini was to report the results to me quickly. I entered the sterile needle biopsy room and put on the white gown that I would come to despise. I laid down on my right side with my left arm up exposing my left side. Putting myself into a meditative state helped me endure the pain of the biopsy like a champ. But when the radiologist reported to me she found cancer in the sentinel node, I lost all composure and let loose a wild scream. Another *strike*.

"I'm going to die, I'm going to die!" I wailed. My turnaround from composure to hysteria was so abrupt that the radiologist put Dr. Sacchini's nurse get on the phone to comfort me.

"No, Lynne, this does not mean you are going to die," she shouted above my sobs. "We have many surviving breast cancer patients who tested positive as you did. But it does mean this will become a chronic illness for you."

Not what I wanted to hear. Another strike to my stability. This was no way to try to enter into the next phase of *coming to terms*; I was not being offered any plateaus from which to compose myself.

The nurse continued to explain: "We and you cannot know the extent of your disease until you have undergone a full mastectomy." *No small lumpectomy for me under the circumstances.* "Several nodes will be taken out during surgery and biopsied right there to find out how many nodes have cancer. Now, I must tell you, this surgery will leave you numb under the arm for every set of nerves cut and prone to infection on the left side of your upper body."

The certain knowledge that I had a chronic cancer condition hit me with renewed disgust and panic. What would I say to my daughter and close friends?

"How bad is it?" they later asked.

I was torn between answering with the medically accurate "I don't know yet" or the more authentic "I don't know, but I am scared I have a fatal disease." It was never clear to me how to respond to friends. I was torn between wanting to immediately call each friend and report the diagnosis, or waiting for more medical clarity about my condition.

The reality of losing a breast and undergoing unspecified further treatments had not yet embedded in my consciousness. It was the fear of going public that first haunted me, the fear of becoming an "other" to my family and loved ones. It took a year before I could bear ordering a "medical alert" bracelet which provides a warning to first responders that I am not to have my blood pressure taken or any needles given on my left side. The bracelet would be the permanent visible mark of my status as having cancer.

We are far removed from the time when Wilber's wife, Treya, underwent draconian and barbaric treatment for her aggressive type of cancer. But treatment is still no walk in the park for any type of cancer. Chemotherapy's side effects have gradually become less stressful on the body. But Wilber is right when he talks about how little doctors are able to speak to *my* prognosis, to *my* survival. I quickly learned to recognize their disclaiming language: "Let's wait and see" or "This will be a chronic disease for you."

As for complementary and alternative methods I later began implementing, and which Sloan-Kettering incorporates in their treatment process on a separate campus, I was very cautious about which ones I selected. Whatever regimen I would be put on after surgery might be lessened in effectiveness by certain alternative ministrations. In addition, many of the websites and books I consulted offered testimonials and anecdotal reports of cures, not double-blind studies. These publications often relied on scare-mongering tactics, where "they" (pharmaceutical companies/doctors/government) "don't want you to know the truth about cancer cures because they will lose money and power." Pre-rational drivel. But yet I certainly planned to carefully incorporate alternative treatments once I figured out how to accomplish a balance.

A pitfall in the *coming to terms* stage is the overabundance of information available thanks to the Internet. Being a researcher by trade and temperament, I spent hours putting together a treatment plan. But it was hard to decipher a pattern in the medical literature, much of which was outdated or from questionable online resources. This roadblock led me to seek more data, which only added to my sense of information overload. I expended countless hours and energy I needed for coping with the trauma of my diagnosis on research, but I couldn't have done otherwise—I craved a sense of power and control over the chaos and endless expanse of white noise confronting me.

At this early moment of my journey, how was I to find meaning and order in this new ordeal? Treya faced an identical dilemma: "Perhaps, after all these years of rather anxiously looking for my life's work, coming down with cancer contained the seeds of this work, if only I could recognize it?" (Wilber, 2000, p. 50)

I too was looking for my life's work in my retirement stage. *What is that all about?* Was I being given a karmic swat on the knuckles to remember how transitory everything is? To just let go of my striving, that at times felt heavy with egoic pressures pushing it, but now was effortlessly and joyfully emerging from within my soul? God bless my support system for helping me through those first days and weeks.

There are many support groups to help those with cancer and I looked up quite a few. I also joined several on-line discussion boards sponsored by such notable organizations as the American Cancer Society. But I also needed people with skills to match my particular needs, and it would require luck and perseverance to find them. It began with my husband who remained close to my side during the entire ordeal; dear friends of 30 year's duration; my closest friend Robin; Lorraine, my integrative therapist; and a woman who reached out from across the country to offer her assistance, Patricia Kay, co-author of a simple yet profoundly informative book entitled *Cell Level Meditation*. Her homeopathic orientation, along with Lorraine's professional and spiritual skills, was the perfect counterbalance to the rigorous scientific perspective of Sloan-Kettering.

I initially turned to the list servers hosted by the various cancer organizations, but following collective misery only left me depressed and unmotivated. One woman had convulsive vomiting from chemo; another came down with lymphedema after her mastectomy. This possible aftereffect of mastectomy, which can be permanently disfiguring, involves an accumulation of lymphatic fluid near the excised lymph nodes. Other women spoke of the discomfort of the post-operative process of the drainage devices they wore at home and which had to be removed after a week or two. I read personal accounts of every possible misery that my sisters endured post-op, and I became depressed and panicky. My husband finally persuaded me to cease following these reports. I stopped, and felt my path lightened when I only concentrated on *my* illness and *my* path toward healing.

The diagnosis of cancer spurred me to dive even deeper into my grief and stress work with Lorraine. All of her techniques were critical to my healing journey, but none more so than the ones that dealt with my mother.

"Pick out a colored pair of felt footprints from the bowl, Lynne," Lorraine prompted. "Put them on the floor to resemble you standing with your mom and dad." I chose medium white ones for me, large red ones for Mom and small blue ones for Dad. I put Mom's footprints directly in front of me and Dad's slightly behind Mom's, as their power dynamic in my life played out.

"Now talk to them, Lynne, from your heart, as to what hurt you yet which you could never speak to them about."

This threw me into a panic, as I never did have the courage to address my hurts and wants directly to them. Then there was my fear that it was blatantly unfair to do this to two people who were now deceased, my beloved parents. So after several false starts, I began to speak to my dad first.

"Why did you sacrifice me to take care of mom's violent mood swings? You called me back from college, you left on the weekends to play golf, or you turned off your hearing aid so that I was left with full control over mom. That was really your job and you didn't do it correctly. I suffered under having her all to myself. That wasn't my job!" I had begun to cry.

"Now your mom, Lynne," Lorraine whispered softly.

Shifting slightly to face the large red footprints, I began, "I know how much you loved me, mom, and how you spent your life taking care of me…"

"What hurt you, Lynne? Get to the hurt and sadness," Lorraine prompted.

"Why did you lay all of the horrible stories of your life and your relatives on me and let me believe that my life would just be a continuation of all of their miseries, because that's what happened! I had a rocky life, thanks to you and your training of me just to serve you and not live for myself, and now I've got cancer. So I won the lousy life lottery!" The anger coiled within my stomach was beginning to unwrap and rise up through my throat.

As I was beginning to drip tears, Lorraine reached into the container and brought out two large white footprints, which she placed behind my mother's; then she shifted the red footprints to face them.

"This is your mother's father, Lynne, Lazarus David, and it is really with him that your mother needs to speak. It is her hurt from her father, the terrible way he treated her and her family, that created the mother who was not able to properly parent you. Let the two of them talk together, let Lazarus ask for forgiveness of his daughter, and then let the two of them resolve their generational issues without you becoming involved."

At another session Lorraine had me visualize my mother and grandmother and all the female ancestors holding my back, while I held onto my daughter Erica's back, and she held onto her son, Adam.

"Your ancestors are supporting you through this trying time, Lynne, and you are responsible for helping future generations by staying alive and teaching them your wisdom." My therapy with Lorraine has continued in a similar vein, with techniques for trauma added when necessary along with the regular "talk therapy." We worked routinely with symbols of all types: stones, quartz, cards, whatever I felt attracted to as a signal of healing.

Patricia Kay came to me at a low time in my treatment. I had been posting to a Yahoo group to which she belonged, and when I posted that my mammogram had been positive for breast cancer, she reached out to me, a complete stranger, to offer her unique gifts. I began to use her professional services through nightly phone calls as she drew me deeper and deeper into the world of my cells, both healthy and cancerous. Cell level meditation, her area of expertise, became my meditation of choice as I learned to breathe into various organs and tissues of my body.

"Cells contain all the intelligence of you, Lynne," she explained. "There are normal cells and now there are mutated, sick, and voracious cancer cells. Can you visualize them both?" Spontaneous images popped into my consciousness that then entwined with my breath to constitute a unique form of meditation. It was a daily and often moment-by-moment fight to keep centered and free from despair. Her words stayed with me: "Sometimes when meditating on the cells, you find that memories pop up that evoke strong emotions. The cells store your life history, Lynne, and yours, for whatever reason, are intense and grief-filled. If you need to talk to that memory, resurrect it, and call out to reconfigure what happened to you on that day during that sad time, do it! Grab the hand of young Lynne and pull her to safety. You will have changed the configuration of your cell memories and functions in that way. Just never stop breathing into your cells, every day, breathe into your organs, tissues—do it all on a cellular level."

Patricia was an invaluable guide through the highest and most minute levels of awareness within my body during this phase of my healing journey. Are she and Lorraine responsible for my cancer-free condition today? Studies do indicate that mental health care and emotional support can help patients like me and my family better manage the cancer and treatments.

My next visit to Sloan-Kettering was to the plastic surgeon, Dr. Mehrara, who showed me pictures of how they would be able to reconstruct a natural looking and feeling left breast from my own stomach tissue—a new breast plus a tummy tuck. Things were beginning to look up that afternoon. They could even create a non-sensitive nipple for the breast. The entire journey would take months, but this light at the end of the cancer tunnel was indeed appealing.

There was no medical reason for me to have reconstructive surgery, since my husband reassured me I would be loved regardless of my post-operative appearance. Many women even opt for a double mastectomy for preventative health reasons. But with large breasts to begin with, I felt it aesthetically and practically beneficial to have my remaining breast reduced and a smaller breast reconstructed to give me a balanced look.

During the mastectomy, Dr. Mehrara would place a silicone shield next to my chest wall. Over time, he would inject saline at the site of the new breast to stretch my skin. When it had reached the cup size I desired, he would take stomach tissue and blood vessels and transplant them under my skin so that my breast would form my tissue again.

By late October 2010, I was beginning to *come to terms* with my new reality. I was in the fourth week after my diagnosis of infiltrating breast cancer and already had had to digest more technical and biological information than I could handle emotionally and cognitively. I was facing a frightening diagnosis, although not terminal (at least at this point). I had a top-notch surgeon and a surgery date of November 4th, more tests that would be somewhat uncomfortable prior to surgery, and then after surgery I would drop off into a liminal space of drugs, pain, discomfort, shocks to my body-mind, and decisions that I would probably make in line with my surgeon's and oncologist's recommendations. I planned to do my usual research, but not to the point of total confusion. Somehow, I was falling into the "she-ro [female hero]" role—an upbeat patient with a little pink ribbon on my blouse and an endless font of laugh-lines.

Before the mastectomy, I fixated on the breast about to be removed. It had nourished my daughter and provided me with great sensual pleasure. I could not accept the dismissive explanation by Dr. Woodward that it was merely an appendage of fatty tissue. Since I was a young woman with developing breasts, I had been so proud of mine; they brought me admiring attention from men even into my sixties. Breasts are perhaps a woman's ultimate sign of desirability, and I was about to lose half of mine.

I poured out my uncertainty to friend Robin: "Until the artificial breast is formed months from now, how will I look in clothes? How can I go out in public? Will I still have cleavage?" Her sister-in-law had just passed away due to small cell lung cancer and thus Robin had no answers to my questions, but at least she could commiserate with me.

"What do prostheses look and feel like, Lynne? Where do you get them? Is there a catalog or place online where you order the shape and size you want?"

I had no answers either, but I certainly had more concerns and questions. The egoic factor of my appearance was trumped by my denial of considering my post-surgical pain. Fear of pain never even came up for me in my therapy, either. I did not want to know; I specifically did not ask my surgeon about using analgesics or opiates, nor did I research this aspect of my treatment. I had no choice but to undergo a radical surgery, so I fled into denial that I would be at the mercy of my body's pain response afterwards. So much for getting in touch with my body.

Surgery did occur as scheduled on November 4th. I repressed any fear responses or thoughts of mortality as I wheeled my suitcase into the surgical area. My husband and I have had the misfortune of spending time in hospitals over our married life, and we pass the pre-operative time being silly and making one another laugh about politics and the weather, or other harmless topics. There were no discussions about possible death on the operating table or last words of love; it was our way of coping with dread and concern, which we

148

both knew underlay the humor. I did not look at my left breast before surgery. I couldn't.

As I awoke from anesthesia, Dr. Sacchini informed me, "Lynne there was some, just a bit, of cancer in the sentinel lymph node, and the two other nodes above it were cancer-free. This is good news, even if it does jump you up to about stage 2a for cancer."

My husband and I were overjoyed. We didn't know at the time the implications of the tiny bit of cancer in the one lymph node. Rick and I thought the rollercoaster had reached its terminus and we could exit the scary ride once I healed.

I did not attempt to touch my left side. It had drains coming out of it into what looked like hand grenades, and was covered in heavy bandaging. Once again, I chose to deny the enormity of what had just occurred. Dr. Sacchini next informed me he would not remain as my treating physician now that the surgery was completed; that role would be filled by a doctor in Basking Ridge, New Jersey, Sloan-Kettering's satellite campus much closer to my home. After a few days in the hospital recuperating and being trained to empty the drains, I returned home.

By 2010, Melissa's mental illness had "burned off," and was completely gone. She emerged from her years of torment as a competent, good-looking professional nurse, devoted mother, and loving wife. I felt honored that she volunteered to care for me after my mastectomy, which she did with all the love and devotion any daughter could have provided for her birth-mother. She monitored the drains, showed me how to do them, explained my medications' side effects, and helped me navigate so that I did not injure my sutures. Our interpersonal healing had taken another huge step forward.

I had been thrown into a new identity by this radical cancer surgery. Foremost, I could no longer deny the absence of my left breast. I needed pain-killers and nursing care for the first few days while I gingerly explored what had been done to me. A hard silicone shield had been placed against my left chest wall to provide a substrate for the injections of skin-stretching saline I would receive every other week for months. There was no longer a nipple or a breast, just sewn tissue with drains protruding. I felt ugly and deformed. I would never be my old self again.

Once I felt well enough to shop, I bought clothes two sizes too large to fit over the bandages and to disguise my imbalanced chest.

Two weeks later I had my first appointment with my medical oncologist in Basking Ridge. In a replica of the main hospital, I discovered that my new doctor was a perky young mother of two boys named Dr. Deena Graham (Dr. G). It was love and trust at first sight. Her wavy hair bounced as she walked, and when she smiled, her eyes disappeared into small slits. Dr. G's nurse, Rose, was a warm, effusive woman I adored the first time I met her. Rose made me feel as though I were her favorite patient, although I witnessed her charm with countless others.

Once Rick and I introduced ourselves to the doctor, Dr. G set about her job of translating the clinical findings from my surgery. She informed me there was a slight possibility cancer cells might have traveled from the sentinel node to my bones or other organs, and therefore I would have to have a nuclear medicine scan of my bone and tissue. I completed the tests in mid-November.

The day before Thanksgiving, Dr. G called me at home.

"Hi, Lynne. I have something to tell you about your tissue scan, but I don't think it's much to worry about." I stopped mid-chop, as I was preparing an appetizer for our family Thanksgiving dinner. Better to stop than to chop off a finger.

"They found a spot on your left lung. Now, I see from your chart you never smoked. I also see you've had asthma, so it could well be old scar tissue."

"What do you think it is, Doctor?" I asked knowing that she could not possibly have a clear idea at this early stage, but still wanting a parental "there, there" and a pat on the head not to worry.

"I really don't think there is anything to concern us, but you will have to get a lung biopsy before we begin chemotherapy on December 6th. Honestly, Lynne you've never smoked, no one in your family smokes; you had no second-hand smoke in your workplace, so it is most probably scar tissue. I wouldn't ruin your holiday over this finding, but we do need to move onto your chemotherapy."

Not chemo. Not the ordeal that Treya wrote about, the bouts of nausea and vomiting, the pain in her bones! Can't you save my life without pumping me full of toxins?

Having chemotherapy or not would ultimately be my choice. I knew I had the right to seek no toxic treatment past surgery, and to rely on complementary or alternative medicine: high doses of vitamin C, ozone treatments with ultraviolet light, immune stimulating treatments, allogenic lymphocyte therapy, laetrile, nutraceuticals, nutritional therapy such as Gerson, plus emotional and spiritual support.

I read through the websites of the more extensively researched complementary and alternative medical methods but got an uneasy feeling. None of them included the latest scientific findings of conventional medicine any more than the conventional methods referenced alternative and complementary sources. I did not wish to leave out any modality that could help me in my fight for life. After weighing my options, I made the decision to embrace both systems as long as they did not conflict or negatively interact.

Strike Two

The well-meaning medical professionals who tut-tutted my feelings of impending doom over first the mammogram and then the needle biopsy left me feeling disillusioned, so Dr. G's reassuring tone left me unconvinced. Could I possibly have lung cancer without having a real risk factor? Am I back to my mother's belief that her family was cursed with bad luck? Wasn't this latest scare proof of that curse or bad karma? No, this could not be happening since I had never smoked or permitted others to smoke near me.

My thoughts immediately turned to Lucinda Stone's recent and horrible death from small cell lung cancer (SCLC) a few months before. I never met Lucinda, who was a friend of a friend, but I heard daily updates about her condition. I heard about the terrible diagnosis, the grim prognosis, and finally the tragic demise of this talented and beautiful young doctor and mother of three small children.

Small cell lung cancer is the most aggressive form of lung cancer and has usually spread to other parts of the body by the time it is diagnosed. Only about 6% of people with this type of cancer are still alive five years after diagnosis, although treatment can often prolong life for six to twelve months, even when the cancer has spread.

SCLC currently accounts for 14% of all lung cancer cases and is associated almost exclusively with people who smoke. In a fearsome new finding, however, Lucinda was considered part of a new cohort of sufferers who never smoked and were in their 40s.

When her surgeon opened her up, he found cancer in tiny dots spread throughout both lungs and in the lining of the lungs, which meant the cancer was inoperable. What must Lucinda have thought as the lightning struck her? What might I learn from those who have struggled before me? Robin said it best in an e-mail to me about my upcoming biopsy:

"You are all these many roles in response to cancer. Yes, perhaps sometimes a victim, and also a warrior, and also a thriver and survivor. What term encompasses all of these? That's the challenge. How to hold that old chaotic mess of different roles and responses and emotions and thoughts about and around the cancer. In addition to the actual physical pain and suffering. It is the Big Mind of Cancer. Many voices."

Many strands of good fortune and bad, as well, I realized.

I went to the lung biopsy with my husband in a state of abject panic and Lucinda's story fresh on my mind. I re-experienced the electrically charged interruption of logical thought. I had random fragments of songs, mind-pictures, and conversation stems all jumbled in my consciousness.

The radiologist at Sloan-Kettering met me as I donned the detested hospital gown and hopped up on the operating table. His arms were crossed and he gazed without cessation at a strange scan illuminated in the operating room.

"This is your scan, Lynne, and to be honest with you, I've shown it around the hospital today to all of my colleagues. No one knows what this is, or has ever seen anything like it before."

My husband and I stared at it as the radiologist prepared for the biopsy. It was impossible to miss the circular shape on my left lobe, looking like a toxic jellyfish. It had a translucent mass with see-through tentacles radiating out and sailing behind. Having seen jellyfish while snorkeling in Hawaii and Australia, it scared the hell out of me, especially since I realized this had to be cancer and it was inside my lung tissue.

152

"You are quite lucky we made this finding, Lynne," he continued. Ah yes, Lynne was *sooo* lucky. But as he explained, it finally got through to me what he meant.

"You see this translucent quality?" he asked as he pointed to the jellyfish.

Yes indeed, we had.

"Well, that means that it would never have been picked up on an x-ray, even as it continued to spread and invade other organs. Only a body scan would have picked this up."

So "yippee!" I had breast cancer?

"The other issue is that this mass is not in an area causing problems or symptoms." Like Lucinda's strange cough prior to her diagnosis, he meant. "You'd have gone on for three years with no x-ray or symptoms hinting at the danger growing inside your lung, until one day, maybe three years from now, you'd have a funny cough and then finally have a scan done. Then they'd tell you it was too late and it was all over."

I felt a wave of relief—lung cancer caught in time by a stroke of great fortune of having had breast cancer and the doctor requiring a body scan!

My husband was ushered out of the operating room. They inserted an IV into my arm to put me to sleep for the biopsy. Feeling woozy and warm, I asked this kindly doctor, "I know you don't know what kind of lung cancer this is, Doctor, but you must have a hunch, don't you? What do you think it is?"

"Small cell lung cancer," he calmly and matter-of-factly responded. And then the lights went out for me.

Cold Sweats and Cold Fear

I returned home after the biopsy to await their conclusions on the jellyfish inside me, and immediately rechecked the medical sites on small cell lung cancer. It was as grim as Lucinda's story had been. I was going to die in 18 months and would definitely be gone before five years.

The biopsy had been conducted on December 3rd, and I spent the following weekend with my newly pregnant daughter and son-in-law at a local restaurant. A smile was frozen on my face as solidly as the snow on the pavement outside. How could I share with them the feeling of impending death that I carried inside, just as Erica had begun to carry life inside of her?

But I had to grit my teeth and smile like a good "she-ro." No need to scare my daughter. She had surprised me on Thanksgiving with the best news any mother could hope for who has been longing for such an event. Counting back, I realized that she had conceived on the day of my mastectomy, and would give birth around July 30th. I had read enough books and articles about stress during pregnancy that the news of my possible impending death would not escape my lips on this gorgeous winter day. Only love and light would emanate from me from now on. Obviously, this put me in conflict with another value of being a role model of transparency. How might I achieve that if I wasn't honest about what I was facing?

The students in my spiritual program were already jarred by my illness and absence, so I was alarmed at the impact my affect might have on my pregnant daughter. I wanted to be a role model and source of authenticity for both the students in my new course and for my own child. I started a public blog on the day of my diagnosis so that I could share with my family, friends and acquaintances what I was experiencing as openly and honestly as I could; but frankly, I found it very difficult to sort through the cultural and personal feelings associated with my diagnosis.

I had my hair cut very short later that day in preparation for my first chemo session scheduled for Monday. My hair was a thick, rich, wavy dark brown with a mind of its own. I heard such dismal stories of how the loss of hair actually hurts, and how it comes out in odd and unsightly clumps that I wanted to have some control over this process.

"Simon," I asked my son-in-law, "how would you like to shave my head tonight?" I had made the quirky decision to permit him to shave it all off once it began to fall out, which happens about 14 days after the first chemo induction. "I remember that I hadn't been very kind to you when you sported a shaved head when we first met. I figure I might lower my karma a few notches if I let you shave all of my hair off." He agreed.

154

So many "shoulds" assaulted me on that frigid winter day dining with my daughter. How authentic and transparent should I be, and to whom did I owe my innermost thoughts? How should I engage with the cultural mandates of having breast cancer? A book called *Pink Ribbon Blues* deals with the cultural examination and understanding of the "illness" of breast cancer. The author, Gayle Sulik, traces the "tyranny" of pink ribbon corporate culture that pushes women into what she feels is an imposed role of a culturally idealized patient who is assertive and boundlessly optimistic while remaining feminine and sexy despite the physical effects of disease and treatment. In contrast, I wanted to walk this walk with as much authenticity as possible, and see into my body, my psyche, my family, and my culture as clearly as possible. Perhaps I could shine a light to guide other women who share a multi-perspectival awareness and who faced similar hurdles in their treatment journey. I realized I would have to continue investing in my own deep self-knowledge if I were to be of use to others and myself.

During the lively lunch conversation that Saturday with my daughter and son-in-law, and amid many funny comments on my upcoming crew cut, I began to get cold sweats. The sweat dripped down my face and back. It came in waves that would not stop, regardless of what medication or powder I tried that evening, although I did not feel feverish. I was obviously scared to death about the first chemo infusion on Monday, I presumed. Fear and anxiety dominated my life all weekend.

Rick drove me to the Basking Ridge treatment center. There were three good things about the center: it was in a beautiful nature park with deer and hawks about; my beloved doctor was there; and her joyous nurse Rose would welcome me and guide me to "that room" with a smile of comfort. If anything could lighten my level of fear, it would be that combination.

This was my first experience with "infusion suites," which is the chic name given to the facility where nurses gowned in HazMat suits and gloves administer the chemotherapy. I was unaware that infusions can last four hours, and there was no food service at the center. Each person or family brought food to last the course of an infusion session, which begins with pre-infusion blood work and culminates in a post-infusion visit to the doctor. I had nothing with me, but I did have 12 pages of printouts from all of the breast cancer blogs about what to eat, wear, throw-up in, suck on, drink, and so on. Every horror story from across the country made it into my compendium, and I was in such a gloomy state that I figured that all of the side-effects of chemo would befall me.

First I had blood work to make sure that I could tolerate the infusion, and then the IV went into my right hand vein. I felt resigned to my sentence, a prisoner walking into the execution chamber with no energy left.

"Here you go, Lynne," chirped the irrepressible Rose, as she swung open the door to the dreaded chemo suite.

As I shuffled forward, like the condemned going to the executioner, Dr. G came rushing towards me waving a fax printout.

"No, Rose, hold it! Hold it! Don't let her go in there! She's got lung cancer!"

Never in history have those words been met with such a wave of relief. I had had my chemo sentence commuted by the doctor, and all it took was a diagnosis of lung cancer. This was incredible in every sense of the word.

Dr. G quickly ushered me into her office after Rose unhooked me from the IV that would have pushed in the pink poison (as I chose to identify the chemotherapy compound) in just a few minutes. We sat down across from one another, with me still feeling a euphoric sense of relief from dodging the chemo bullet. Granted, this was not a standard reaction to learning that I had *two* major cancers.

"Is it small cell lung cancer?" I blurted out. By now I was in emotional and physical overload. The cold sweats poured down my face and onto the remaining breast tissue; my energy had abandoned me and any feeling of hope for my future became academic rather than personal. This was not the time for polite comments about her children; this was a fight for my life with *two* villains now snapping at my heels.

"No, we don't know what kind it is, but we do know it is not small cell. The problem here," she continued without permitting me to jump in with another explosion, "is that we don't know yet if this
156

is a primary cancer or your breast cancer having metastasized to the nearby lung tissue, and that has an effect on survival rates."

"OK, tell me what you think this lung cancer is, and how long I have to live." I was alert now and ready to hear the unvarnished truth. The fact that chemo was no longer being discussed had put me in a better mood.

"Lynne, I honestly believe this is breast cancer that has metastasized into your lung. That means that your life span is about five years. But we will not stop trying, and there are new discoveries every day."

And Martians might come to visit me tonight. My mood turned sour once again. What was the use of five years, I thought rather ungenerously? In the face of an 18-month diagnosis, who wouldn't plead for five full years, I realize now. I collapsed into myself once again, and began shivering. My pregnant daughter would deliver a child who would hardly remember her grandma. Five years—the same amount of time Treya had after her breast cancer was discovered.

But the doctor interrupted my fatalistic reverie with instructions: "Your next step, Lynne, will be to see our lung surgeon and schedule surgery. Then we'll know more and I can tell you about our next steps."

Her glorious smile had come out of the shadows and I was feeling better, yet still cold, as I exited the building to inform my husband of this new lightning strike. Unfortunately for Rick, I bounded into the car with a smile on my face, which led to massive confusion when I informed him about my lung cancer. Once again, I felt as though I was on a rollercoaster. I could attempt to find a better metaphor, but there is nothing more apropos to describe the stomach-wrenching highs and lows of cancer.

Strike Three

The cold sweats continued all week and I noticed that the area that would someday house my new breast was getting pinker than the surrounding skin. Six days later I awoke with a fever, and the area where the surgeon had patched up my removed breast had turned a bright, nasty shade of red. This could not be a good turn of events. As the day unfolded, the red patch swelled larger. I knew enough to call my plastic surgeon at 11:00 that night. By then I was scared. The cold sweats turned into a burning fever and the swelled, red skin area looked as though it were creating its own mad and frightening breast.

The doctor told me to pack a bag and rush over to the Sloan-Kettering emergency room in Manhattan for what would be a minimum of a three-day stay. I had cellulitis, he explained, and off Rick and I drove into the cold dark night.

Cellulitis is a common bacterial infection that lodges in tissue beneath the skin, and is most commonly caused by *Staphylococcus* and *Streptococcus* bacteria. Recall the insertion of the silicone breast shield next to my chest wall prior to the saline infusion to stretch my skin; it did not take a brilliant person to figure out what I had, and how I had contracted it. The treatment would be three days on IV antibiotics.

Unbeknownst to me at the time, Rick had driven home in tears; he suspected that this condition would prove to be far worse than anticipated.

And it was.

After five days on the strongest IV antibiotics possible, the infection kept progressing. My left breast area looked like a fuchsia-colored water balloon, and my fever was on the march to higher numbers every day. The doctor and his staff were worried, and he called for emergency surgery late that afternoon. I could not wait. I was so sick and just wanted to get well enough to find out what would happen to me next.

Dr. Mehrara performed the emergency surgery. He discovered that it was the breast shield that kicked off the infection; in other words, the infection had started deep in my tissues and worked its way out toward my skin. He told me he flushed a quart of pus out of me, and then joked that it was the 20th grossest surgery he'd ever performed. My dark sense of humor took this as quite a compliment, and I repeated it to my friends. Three more days and I could go home.

On the day after this emergency surgery, as I was awakening early that morning feeling as though I were hallucinating, a thin man

158

appeared to be sitting in a chair by my bed. As my vision and consciousness cleared, I saw he was real.

"Hello, Lynne, I'm Dr. Rizk and I will be your lung surgeon."

His name appeared pretty appropriate for his specialty.

"No, this is not small cell lung cancer," he responded to my first coherent query. Good news!

"It's called BAC, or bronchioloalveolar carcinoma. This type of lung cancer occurs in never-smokers like you for reasons we don't understand yet, as well as in smokers, and it's found in women to the same extent as men. I'm going to get rid of it all for you via surgery, and I believe you will be a suitable candidate for arthroscopic surgery. We'll do some lung tests and then you'll rest up for about a month before we take care of this latest problem. You'll leave surgery with three little puncture wounds on your back. Not a bad deal."

Talk about a joyous day! I would leave my left lobe behind and only have three small bandages. I could keep my thick brown hair since no chemo is recommended for the lung cancer I had. I saw a return to my normal life appearing before my eyes. I wouldn't ever have to undergo chemo for either of the cancers, I thought. I would have a pain-free lung cancer surgery that would rid my body of the horrid scourge, and be able to return to the classroom to revive my program. I could rejoin my life now in progress. At least that was my mental plan that day. Things played out quite differently.

The next time I entered Sloan-Kettering, I would be on the Sixth Floor with other lung cancer patients. I explained to my floor nurse that I would be returning in a month for my lung cancer surgery, which was at Stage Ia, and she immediately teared up. She had not met anyone with early and treatable lung cancer before. I realized I would be among very sick cancer patients next time.

With life coursing through me and denial of negative possibilities coming back on line, I returned home for the month before my final surgery.

My outlook was that I had dodged the worst cancer bullets.... for now.

Part 2

COMING TO TERMS

CHAPTER TEN

The Aftermath

By January 7, 2011, I had moved beyond the initial *lightning strikes* and began moving more comfortably toward the phase of the healing cycle I called *coming to terms*. My lung surgery was scheduled for 11:00 A.M. Monday morning, January 10th. I had met with Sloan-Kettering personnel that previous Monday, and all day Wednesday I was worn out from the pre-operative medical procedures. I did find out from the nurse that researchers are discovering more and more Stage Ia lung cancers from accidental findings on scans and x-rays.

I also felt "growly," which I characterized as a combination of frustration, disgust, annoyance, and a desire to remain just where I was in the safe cocoon of my home. The three plantings outside of my kitchen door, the upright and proud green and blue spruces with the tan drooping feathers of the ornamental grasses between them, were decorated by the recent snow in precisely the way I desired, and they offered their beauty to me at every glance. The firs wore shrugs of puffy snow, while the trees behind them stood tall with icing on every branch.

Deer, possum, raccoon, cat, and skunk tracks created intricate embroideries of paw and hoof prints in the snow up to the feeding platters we set out for them for their winter picnic. My sweet little white puppy, Chloe, stood erect at the door hoping to be incited by a fleeing or teasing grey or black squirrel, although I half believed that she woofed for the sheer exuberance of hearing her own voice.

I mostly felt resentful that my meditation and my contemplation in the nest of my home was to be disrupted by a return to Sloan-

161

Kettering. I'd be back amidst the busy-ness of the hospital, the every-three-hour vitals check, the lack of tranquility and of self-direction about every bodily function.

By the next day I noticed this "growliness" had permitted suffering to re-enter my life. "If we get caught in our notions and concepts, we can make ourselves suffer and we can also make those we love suffer," says Buddhist philosopher Thich Nhat Hanh. By stepping aside from my ego I began to witness what I was doing to myself. At first I had been in a state of bliss while resting in the moment in my beloved kitchen; but by choosing to switch out of the moment to my impending surgery that Monday, all of that bliss dissipated and was replaced by a version of suffering, which manifested as *agita*. By leaping forward to the unknowable tomorrow I came unmoored from the moment.

I had to admit to myself in a somewhat self-deprecating manner that freedom, peace, and joy in the present moment were the most important things I could have, especially under these times fraught with possible lethal peril. I would have to concentrate on a more awakened understanding of impermanence, or I would ruin any possible moment of happiness. By putting conditions on my happiness of the moment, by leaping forward to the pain of the next moment or the next tomorrows, I destroyed the momentary bliss I felt in my kitchen.

Along with the anxiety over pain and prognosis, I harbored some very pedestrian gripes about my coming hospital stay. There would be the constant activity of the hospital staff, the annoyance with roommates and their families which had led me to explode during my last stay. I had to allow these factors to function without placing conditions or fears or anger upon them. I mulled over how I would digest the serious and mundane issues as they arose, rather than projecting them into my present.

January 10th came and I fairly bounded up the steps at Sloan-Kettering. *What, me worry?* I was home free. I smiled and joked through the pre-operational tests and cheerfully slipped into the surgical gown. They had to administer an IV and then an epidural, they informed me. I kissed Rick goodbye and let them wheel me into the operating room while I mentally predicted the procedure would be as minimally painful as a visit to the dentist.

But the IV insertion caused me to scream louder and with more pain than any of the other two surgeries. Apparently, the harsh antibiotics they had administered into my veins to combat the cellulites had so irritated my veins that I could not bear another IV, no matter where they inserted it on my right arm or hand.

When I awoke, Rick and Dr. Rizk were there. The doctor had good and bad news for me.

"I'm so glad to tell you we took out the entire cancer in the left lower lobe, and you are free of lung cancer as far as we can tell, Lynne." His then lowered his voice.

"But when I entered your back to perform the surgery arthroscopically, I would have had to go through the area where you had the cellulites infection. I could not risk pushing any residual bacteria into your lungs, so I had to perform a thoracotomy. You will be placed on heavy pain meds because this procedure is the most painful of all cancer surgeries. But you're going to be just fine."

Pain. Health. I'd been given both.

I began to understand what my surgery entailed. My ribs had been spread, nerves cut and damaged, and muscles moved; I had tubes exiting me again for drainage. I was given a pillow to press against my chest whenever I had to cough or take a deep breath. Without heavy pain medication, I screamed with every move. That first night I was prescribed a heavy painkiller that I did not tolerate well. As I am a happy drunk, it turned out that I was a happy over-medicated patient. Sometime around midnight I began calling to the nurses telling them to prep me for going home.

"I'm ready to go home now," I sing-songed repeatedly to the nurse, the doctor, and the cleaning lady. I was a kindly patient, but my misapprehension of what my condition was worried the staff.

"Lynne," asked the charge nurse, "who is the president?"

"Oh," I cooed back, "I can't remember his name, but he's a very nice man."

"OK, you need a different pain medication," he concluded.

I continued to smile idiotically and repeat the refrain that I was ready to leave.

I finally did get released after four more days and recuperated at home on the correct dosage of oxycodone and oxycontin. I never felt high as a result of this combination, just able to tolerate the pain better. I screamed for several weeks when I changed positions, but I resolved to move through the pain with few complaints. After all, I was at an end of my travails. Or so I thought.

Back with my oncologist in Basking Ridge at the end of January 2011, we met to discuss what treatment would follow my three serious surgeries in three months. I sauntered into her office, with feet barely touching the ground. Two serious cancers vanquished and a possibly fatal infection subdued. Now was the time for her to congratulate me and send me on my way to lead a healthy and recovered life. After we shared notes on her two sons and Erica's pregnancy, she got down to business.

"Lynne, there is absolutely no doubt in the studies that you need chemo in order to beat your breast cancer. With it, your chances of recurrence fall to 17%. Without chemo, your chances of recurrence are over 26%. We need to start soon, and the second week of February marks the latest time chemo will be effective."

I began to cry for the first time. This meant I still had cancer; it was lurking inside me and could launch a training camp somewhere inside my body with the intention of spreading out recruiting cells to once again form masses and destroy my life.

"I think it is a course you would want to take with your daughter pregnant and you with professional plans to pursue," she recited calmly.

I am impressed by statistics, those anchors upon which we hang our fragility. And with the odds heavily weighted in favor of good outcomes for me statistically, why would I cry in frustration and rage? Because the treatment meant more pain. Hair loss. Feeling sick all the time. Bone pain. I recited my fears to Dr. G and continued to cry; since she had never seen me in tears, she called the social worker to speak with me, but it made no difference.

I recalled all of the horror-filled blogs, the books detailing the day-to-day misery of women on chemo, and I knew I faced a future of specific suffering that was well known in this treatment. Tears do not come easy to me, so my gushing signaled to loved ones and

164

friends the bravura I had demonstrated during three hospitalizations had disappeared. For all intents and purposes, I had been hit by another *lightning strike* and my *coming to terms* had evaporated. This next part of my journey struck me perhaps irrationally as far more frightening than my previous cancer treatments.

I continued to cry for two weeks and to seek out friends who might accept my terror while holding me lovingly in their embrace. On Valentine's Day I went into the dreaded chemo suite where the first half of the chemical treatment regimen would be administered. As I peeked inside, I was greeted by what looked like a modern office complex with transparent partitions creating small cubicles each with a luxurious leather reclining chair, a visitor's chair, and a TV set. I was escorted to room number 14, where I was asked if I wanted a warmed-up, hand-knitted comforter to ward off the chill of the room.

There are several stages to the infusion process. First I was given steroids, then an antihistamine, and then six heavy pink vials were added to the IV. Denial of what was occurring was my ally. My husband and I watched "Judge Judy" and other TV shows on the monitor by my reclining chair as I swaddled myself in the comforters provided by volunteers. I slept for part of the long session. I refused to permit my mind to focus on all of the unknown side-effects I would have to endure after leaving the infusion suite.

Upon returning home I began a course of frequent injections in my stomach, several anti-nausea drugs, and countless pills to be taken in precise order. I couldn't eat or drink normally and lost eleven pounds in two weeks. The simple solution was to increase the anti-nausea drugs, which helped. Nevertheless, my appetite changed radically as did my ability to swallow any liquid. Everything tasted like oil. Only after numerous trials did I come up with the solution of drinking watermelon juice and privileging white foods.

My regimen was to have an infusion once every two weeks. The standard response was to feel weak and terrible the first week, bounce back the second week, and then repeat for two months. Yes, there was nausea, bone pain that kept me from sleeping, and hair that hurt as it withered and fell out in clumps. Indeed, hair fell out all over my body: pubic, legs and arms, eyebrows and eyelashes. I read online catalogues to see how best to disguise my situation. I did purchase a wig that looked so much like my own hair that few friends knew what was going on underneath. I then got back some of my sense of humor and purchased several wigs in different styles so that I could sport a different style on different days: "Sandy" when I felt flirtatious, "Brenda" when I wasn't feeling happy, and "Aubrey" for the go-to-hell blues periods. Expensive or cheap, every wig proved to be sweaty and itchy. After a few weeks I threw them in the back seat of my car and went "commando." Rick mistook a tall bald man for me from behind in one store. Thinking he'd surprise me, he wrapped his hands around the man's midsection and whispered, "Hello, gorgeous."

In mid-March, I spiked a high fever that I was sure was a sinus infection. The only odd thing was the large round red painful "ball" under my right forearm that I presumed was a sprained muscle. I was not permitted to lift anything heavy with my left arm due to the lymph node surgery and the fear of limphedema. So I had toted all heavy bags with my right arm.

Off we went to the local emergency room where I was outfitted with a surgical mask and put into an isolated corner of the hospital to keep my compromised immune system from coming into contact with infectious patients. Indeed, for the entire five months I endured chemo, I did not enter a shopping mall, attend religious services, or see a movie.

The nurse had suspicions about the red lump on my arm and called a vascular specialist. He confirmed it was a blood clot, which breast cancer patients have a tendency to develop. Having the clot in my arm was far better than in the leg since it is not likely to split off and move to the lungs with dire consequences.

After three day's hospitalization for the sinus infection and the clot, I returned home. To prevent another clot, I was put on Coumadin (warfarin), which is, in effect, rat poison. It keeps blood from any type of injury, internal or external, from clotting, and therefore I ran the risk of bleeding to death either from eating leafy green vegetables, which inhibit the effectiveness of warfarin, or from a cut or injury. So now I was on toxic chemotherapy agents plus rat poison, and all this was healthy for me? Plus, I could no longer enjoy veggies, which had been a mainstay during bouts of nausea. I felt like a toxic dump.

After two months on the first half of my chemical cocktail I was switched to the next drug regimen. My reaction to it was far different than the first half: on my first infusion I slept for 19 hours. Dr. G altered its administration by having me come in weekly for three months. I finally found some time to reflect on what had been an intense medical journey, with all of the protocols to follow and the ups and downs of the treatment process.

I made it through to the other side and transformed myself with the help of the Integral model. I had gone through therapy and deep grief work with Lorraine and worked spiritually on the cellular level with Patricia. The problem of inheriting some of my mother's disordered thinking continued to stall a complete recovery. Her vacillation between pre-rational and transcendent ways of looking at reality was among my earliest recollections and therefore one of the hardest parts of my emotional and cognitive self to "re-parent." When I was five years old and being tucked into bed, I hunkered under my covers all self-satisfied. Then the wondering began...

Wait a minute. Mommy tells me I come from the most special family. But all the other mommies are telling their little boys and girls the same thing. Mommy says being Jewish is the best thing to be. But all the other mommies are telling their children they have the best religion to be. So who is right? Aren't all those mommies right too?

At that young age I could not resolve the idea that "If everybody's right, then everybody's wrong." Until I could find a concept of the world that separated out my mother's more embracing statements from the fantasy and egoic posturing, I could never feel supported and assured that the world functioned as my developing sensibilities presumed. I never did feel safe in the world my mother created for me. I was stuck with her confused understandings at some times, but struck by her utter brilliance and out-of-the-box consciousness at others.

My mother combined brilliant creativity with blatant pathology. How was I to account for her extraordinary abilities while under hypnosis and when in her trance-like states? She was obviously channeling something profound when engaged in writing or

167

working on her artistic projects. Ineffable beauty came through her, but so did her psychologically abusive behavior toward me. Was there a connection between her complex of creative abilities and her mental challenges? I needed to become clear at last about the reality I faced, but without my mother's insertion of her magical thinking and pathological intrusions. How could I fight these cancers and move through to recovery laden with this heavy emotional baggage? I turned once again to the Integral model's most basic component: the four quadrants. The quadrants helped me *come to terms* with my health challenges devoid of pre-rational, magical thinking.

Quadrants

In many ways, the four quadrants are the core of Integral Theory. The quadrants dictate that there are at least four perspectives, or ways that we can see the world:

1. The *subjective* comes directly from my feelings, ideas, thoughts
2. The *intersubjective* comes from your and my culture
3. The *objective* exists as concrete realities within my body
4. The *interobjective* exists within systems as rules and protocols that must be honored by nations, economic systems, and businesses

In addition, the quadrants have two axes: inside/outside and individual/collective. To be aware of an inside, I must be aware of an outside; to be aware of an individual entity, I must acknowledge there is a collective/plural as well.

"I" have an emotion (e.g., I am scared of having a mastectomy). "My" emotion of being scared has a corresponding brain state as part of the exterior physical organism of my "It." We can scan my physical fear, my *objective* interior state, by seeing which parts of my brain light up when I am feeling fear after the cancer diagnosis, which is a *subjective* interior state. This state can be treated with medication so that I feel relief from the anxiety that is registering both emotionally and physically.

Then there are group *subjective*, cultural beliefs held by the "We" about the causes of disease. Did growing up in the late 1950's in a Southern culture cause me to be too compliant a daughter? Did I not push back strongly those who harassed me? Many of my friends act strongly enough against those in my groups who harassed me?. Still others felt my high stress levels led to the cancers. I tended to agree with this cultural viewpoint.

The "Its" can be recognized as our legal system or medical protocols in the group *objective* exterior state. Sloan-Kettering recommends certain medications, surgeries, and treatments based on double-blind studies reported on in prestigious medical journals. Lie detector test results cannot be used in New Jersey courts, an aspect of an inter-objective exterior state about their truth. Our courts believe the results are objectively unreliable and have made rules against their admission.

Wilber argues that no one can be 100% wrong about their perspective, and therefore all perspectives must be right, at least partially. But wouldn't this just cause me even more confusion and grief by having to place every treatment idea on the table? Quite the contrary. The universe allowed these many treatment practices to arise in the first place, and the Integral model finds a home for each of these as *partial* truths. All modes of inquiry are an important piece of the overall puzzle in Integral Theory, which forced me to adopt or adapt various perspectives.

If I were to believe in just the alternative and complementary components of treating breast cancer, and reject the objectively verified treatments, I would be left with the following contradictory and possibly harmful choices:

1. Pray the cancer away
2. Use herbs and indigenous treatments alone
3. Enter into a religious or spiritual tradition or community that has methods for dealing with physical illness

4. Undergo psychotherapy to figure out why I had given myself cancer
5. Receive unconventional treatments that my doctors did not want me to know about
6. Scour the Internet for testimonials about folks whose cancers had been cured and adopt their methods

These approaches utilized separately or in random groupings "wouldn't be integral" because:

> "The whole point about any truly integral approach is that it touches bases with as many important areas of research as possible before returning very quickly to the specific issues and applications of a given practice." (Schlitz, p. *xx*)

When I looked at these alternatives I saw they did have commonalities as well as differences:

1. Some dealt with a way for me to inquire about emotions, thoughts, religion, or spiritual practice from the **individual interior** mode of inquiry, involving "I."
2. Others dealt with culturally accepted beliefs about sickness and healing, about how best to heal, and what beliefs hinder or aid our recovery. These **collective interior** beliefs are what constitute a sense of "We," because there are multiple communities to which we might belong.
3. When considering my choice of treatments, I included which physical parts were affected and what the side effects of each might be. I used an **individual exterior** mode of inquiry, or "It."
4. Finally, I would also be forced to deal with **collective exterior** systems of bureaucratic rules and established medical practices, the "Its." Even "praying away the cancer" can have very specific protocols and demands that only certain prayers be administered.

I could engage in the six activities I listed above so long as I could account for their presence within each of the four categories, which would mean that I'd "hit" all bases of my lived experiences.

The six activities do not constitute a perfect integral approach to healing. None that I mentioned are rational approaches to my medical challenge that come from science and reason, from rigorous double-blind testing and peer review. Others do not rise to the level of acceptable rational scientific verifiable approaches to my cancers; these pre-rational belief systems are based on myth and magic in that they were acceptable to humanity prior to the age of science and reason. A few others are trans-rational, in that they reach for an understanding that is high in spiritual sophistication and development.

With the advent of integrative and Integral Medicine, doctors and their patients are trying to redress the pull toward exclusively scientific treatment approaches. Unfortunately, some feel there is no real "truth" to science. They rely exclusively on their individual or cultural interpretations of cancer diagnosis and treatment. This push/pull is neither complete nor balanced. But hope lies around the corner as long as humans continue to develop deeper understandings of who they are in relation to the universe in which they find themselves. A host of research studies have validated the mind-body connection where both doctors and patients are permitted to look at emotional factors as impacting healing (Schlitz, p. xvi).

How was I to figure out a balanced approach to my healing? What was my personal truth about the various steps I might take? Confused from my earliest memory by my mother's alternating between profound and loving insight, and psychotic breaks, I needed something to help me with my choices of treatment. "Lynne Donna, only your mother knows what is right," was the refrain that had circumvented my adoption of my own standards. Her advice contained part truth and part pathology. I'd have to begin teasing apart the good and the true from partial and perhaps pre-rational magical beliefs like "the curse of the Greenbergs" which would leave me hopeless. But if everything had an aspect of truth within it, then how could I make health decisions?

I applied four different tests as truth claims to each of the choices that confronted me. This would assist me in the course of action I wished to take when dealing with my illness. Instead of being limited to an objectivist or scientific test to every question in my life, I would have the breadth, depth, and nuance to assess each choice in a manner that was congruent with its position in what I saw as reality. The four quadrants were essential in helping me decide the next steps.

I proceeded to "go around the quadrants," filling in my responses to the "I" to "It" to "We" to "Its." This process made it simpler by anchoring my choices to the four overarching orienting generalizations as seen in the chart below:

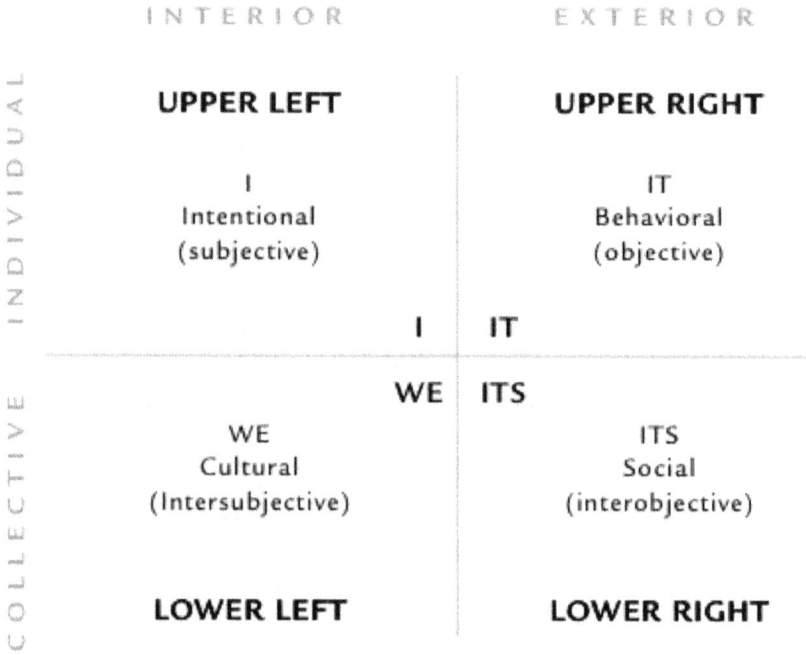

	INTERIOR		EXTERIOR
INDIVIDUAL	**UPPER LEFT** I Intentional (subjective)	I | IT WE | ITS	**UPPER RIGHT** IT Behavioral (objective)
COLLECTIVE	WE Cultural (Intersubjective) **LOWER LEFT**		ITS Social (interobjective) **LOWER RIGHT**

Figure 1. The Four Quadrants of Integral Theory.

Once I drew my own chart, I could begin filling in my thoughts and truths regarding my health issues:

"I," or my self (Upper Left): "My extremely stressful life and negative emotions have made me ill. If I believe that all will be well and abide by my list of health affirmations, then I shall become and stay healthy."

"It," or my body (Upper Right): "As long as I eat a certain diet, take special supplements, or begin an intense body practice, nothing further need be done to heal me."

"We," or our culture (Lower Left): "I will join a support group at my house of worship, and through our joint beliefs I shall be healed."

"Its," or medical systems (Lower Right): "I read that there is a procedure in Germany/Mexico/Costa Rica where a medicine unavailable in United States' hospitals is said to cure cancer. If it cured one person, it can cure me too."

Each of these perspectives reflected some aspect of my health beliefs, but none of them alone would keep me healthy or get me well. I can exercise and diet as much as I like ("It" body), but if I break my leg I'll need a well-equipped hospital and surgeon to help me heal ("Its" system). If as a society we don't believe in the value of healthcare for all (our cultural "We"), then the hospital will be run down and there will be no individuals willing and able to have the motivation ("I") to train as doctors and nurses. It doesn't matter how much I believe in my own good health ("I" Self); positive intentions won't work unless I do something about my physical health and monitor my nutritional behaviors. However healthy I am as an individual won't make a difference if I live in the center of a polluted city.

So I went around the quadrants figuring out how my health interacted with my being-in-the-world. From that point I could select the actions and choices that met my personal truth claims. From each perspective I am able to make assertions about the quality of my actions:

- **Self**: I value the truthfulness and integrity of my thoughts, emotions, states of being, stage of consciousness, and personality type.

- **Body**: I value the physical behavior and vitality of my body. Right now my left arm is hurting me near the incision site, and I must consult with my oncologist rather than ignore it out of fear that it might be a serious complication.

- **Culture**: I want mutual understanding within the medical and healing culture to which I most closely affiliate, including my friends.

- **Systems**: I seek to operate inside the rules, systems, and medical or treatment protocols, particularly those set by Sloan-Kettering.

How I Came To My Heath Decisions

Body

The Upper-Right quadrant is governed by factual knowledge and the language of science, biology, chemistry, physics, immunology, and the domains that treat me as a "biomachine." I value the integrity of my own body and do not want it tampered with more than is absolutely necessary. When Dr. Woodward advised me of my treatment options, I understood she would be dealing with me as a physical object. I needed some way to assess, to weigh, to discern what would be in my best interest as a physical treatment.

I needed to establish my personal, subjective belief about my body by looking at my physical behaviors and how my body had been working. I could make decisions about my care and treatment by paying attention to this bodily, somatic sense. I knew I harbored very strong preferences in regard to my body:

- I did not want my breast taken off; I would campaign for a lumpectomy
- I was afraid of the damage that chemotherapy and radiation would do to my body
- I would take herbs and homeopathic remedies to complement the other procedures to rid my body of cancer cells
- I would continue eating an organic diet

- I would use meditation during any future painful procedures as I did during the needle biopsy

Thoughts and Emotions

The Upper-Left quadrant represents my thoughts, emotions, and experiences shape my choices and actions. This is where my self-sense resides, my sense of being an individual entity in the world. All of the busy-ness of the mind resides here, as well as what we know and what spiritual people call the soul.

I had to decide rather quickly where I would be treated. I believed where I went for treatment would govern the chances of a "good outcome." I believed the gold standard for cancer treatment in the northeastern United States was Sloan-Kettering, but that was the one facility that made me shudder because it was also the place where I felt that people went to die of cancer. At least that was what I had seen over the decades----people checked into Sloan and then passed away soon afterwards.

My fear dissipated after the second call from my husband while still in the doctor's office at Heights Cancer Center. Although my doctor was the finest breast surgeon locally, my husband's close friend urged us to see his wife's surgeon at Sloan, whom he claimed had saved his wife's life. To validate this emotional, intentional switch, I turned once again to the Integral model and weighed my truth of this claim. My husband's friend and his wife had lived their entire lives in New York and selected only the best healthcare providers for them. Their decision coincided with what I had read about Sloan's national ranking and thus it passed the trustworthiness test for me. Compare this to the conversation I had with the massage therapist who claimed his efforts alone could cure the cancerous mass in my left breast. Although I am sure he was sincere, I did not know him, and had no sense of his trustworthiness. The same was true for the friend who warned me that I need rely on good thoughts alone.

I began to consider what my thoughts and emotions revealed:

- I was afraid I was going to die at the very moment when a grandchild was gestating within my beloved daughter.

- I would accept treatment that would promise me the best chance of not dying. To be honest, I held this lightly since I had grave qualms about permitting radiation treatment, and chemotherapy scared me to my core.
- I had been diagnosed with generalized anxiety after the two years of harassment and scapegoating by the superiors at my school. I did not want this stress to continue.
- I had repeated nightmares dating back to that time, and believed that the stress had contributed to my cancer.
- I would continue with the talented and intuitive integrative healer with whom I had been working since 2008.
- I wanted to forgive the three men who harassed me at work so that my thoughts and emotions were as positive as possible.
- I gathered my closest friends around me as my "tribe" and asked for their support.
- I was worried about the "I always have bad luck with health issues" thoughts and needed a way to expunge them.
- Do affirmations, guided imagery, and meditation work with cancer?
- Would I have a good rapport with my doctors, or would they be impersonal and prone to treat me as just a physical object?
- How depressed would I become as it sunk into my consciousness that I was in a fight for my life?
- I wondered if I would actually comply with the treatment and medications—would I go through with chemotherapy and radiation if my medical team recommended this path?

One of the first questions I was asked during each screening is whether I have been under severe stress recently, which was cause enough for a rueful laugh. I had just been stripped of my safe workplace, my area of rewarding connection with my students. I had been berated and defamed, my accomplishments ignored.

In therapy, Lorraine had me deal with the three men at my

school by having me visualize them sitting on her couch. I "saw" into each man's fears and weaknesses until the charge I felt toward them dissipated. This enabled me to reclaim my unique self. I had been a good teacher who could actually midwife transformation in my students. Being a parent loved by her child and thriving in the midst of chaos gave me justification that I had standing in the world. Being a cherished wife for over forty years reopened my sense of value to others. There had been times during traumatic events over the decades when I wished my life could end. In my thirties I had actually figured I'd be satisfied living until I turned 60, and then I'd be freed from this place of endless nightmares. My latest traumatic experience had rekindled that thought. It proved to be hard work replacing those negative emotions with the will to fight for my life.

Now consider this "connect the dots" irony, this karmic joke: the week that my daughter ceased taking the pill in an attempt to get pregnant was the very day I returned home from surgery with a breast removed, the same breast she suckled upon eagerly as a little one, that gave her nourishment, protection, and love. I had a superb reason to stay alive now. I wanted to see her give birth; I wanted to be strong and healthy to play with my grandchild(ren) because I would be a marvelous grandma.

My dark thoughts were also lessened when I researched how meditation could help me with the feared pain from any chemo treatment I might have to endure (Kyung-Eun Choi et al., 2011). Recent studies have shown that meditators exhibit significantly greater tolerance to pain—this was shown not to be due to a placebo effect—and that meditation is an effective technique for alleviating pain, leading to the release of endorphins. The *Journal of Neuroscience* reported that meditators demonstrated a 40% reduction in pain intensity and 57% reduction in pain unpleasantness; in comparison, administration of morphine relieved pain by 25% (Zeidan et al., 2011, p. 215).

One study I read highlighted the danger of believing that healing occurs in one quadrant or one aspect at a time. Researchers Marja Verhoef and Andrea Mulkins researched whether every form of life had been organized for optimum functioning and wellness. They believed that if there was interference in this balance of life force energy, then the organism lost its innate balance, and illness resulted. Verhoef and Mulkins hypothesized that healing occurs as a progression beginning at Level 1, the physical level. Once this level is healed, the individual can deal with Level 2 healing, the energetic level, where balance and wholeness is restored. Then on to Level 3, the mental/emotional arena; then on to the subconscious of Level 4, and finally the spiritual balance of Level 5 might be achieved. The authors were unable to prove their hypothesis, however, and concluded that:

> Healing is not a homogeneous experience... Healing experiences were different for everyone as they were shaped by participants' life experiences and the meanings they attach to people and events....The trajectory of healing was perceived to be in a constant state of flux....As one participant said, "I think it is an ongoing process, I don't think there's a definite start and a stop or end to it. I think it is continuous." (Verhoef & Mulkins, p. 233)

The four phases of the healing cycle I experienced tracked the progression from the body narrative, to interior witnessing mind, to exterior calm-abiding mind, and culminated with a feeling of connection with all being. In my experience, these phases cycled with the changes in my condition. In that sense, healing is an ongoing process until the traumatic changes cease for that disease.

The more frequently I cycled through the phases, the easier it became to segue from one to the next. I held onto my memory of being united with all creation, known as unitive consciousness, and replayed it in my mind to comfort myself when I was in the midst of an emotional storm from the effects of a new upheaval in my diagnosis. When a *lightning strike* hit me, I knew I would need time and techniques to muddle my way through until I came to that gap, that all-important cessation of thought and busy-ness, when I could open up to the next unfoldment of the healing cycle. Within that gap and all subsequent gaps I aimed to open up and honor the mystery that permeates life. I did not lay down a firm track as to how to achieve *coming to terms*, for I knew the manner in which I would relate to the next stage of my healing shared broad similarities with the last cycle, but was imbued with its own mystery and grace.

In an attempt to deal with the lightning strike of my needle biopsy, I clung to any relevant statistics, which, as I have noted, put me emotionally at ease. In fact, the first time I met with Dr. Sacchini I asked him about the survival rates for a lumpectomy versus a mastectomy. I was emotionally persuaded and cognitively reassured by his initial calculations. He presumed I did not have a cancerous lymph node, and therefore death rates after a lumpectomy were 5% to 8%, whereas after a mastectomy they were 4%. It wouldn't matter much to my long-term survival which surgical procedure I underwent. So I figured I wouldn't have to lose my breast, I thought. Very good news. I trusted him.

Would I need any type of systemic treatment, I wondered. The Mayo Clinic maintains an excellent website that deals with cancer and the common myths surrounding its treatment, including these two:

Myth: Everyone with the same kind of cancer gets the same kind of treatment.

Truth: Your doctor tailors your treatment to you. What treatment you receive depends on where your cancer is, whether or how much it has spread, and how it's affecting your body functions and your general health.

Individualized treatment is an exciting development. Drug regimens are tailored to reflect and align with the way each person's body processes chemotherapy treatment, which is why genetic testing was conducted on my particular cancer cells.

Myth: Everyone who has cancer has to have treatment.

Truth: It's up to you whether or not you want to treat your cancer. You can decide this after consulting with your doctor and learning about your options. (Mayo Clinic)

A person with cancer might choose to forgo treatment if he or she has a very slow-growing cancer, as my aunt and mother did. They both had their tumors removed when they were in their 90s during outpatient surgery, and then took tamoxifen thereafter. Both women suffered from other serious medical conditions, which was another reason that they delayed treatment as long as they could. A final reason not to be treated is if the individual has a late-stage cancer where no treatment would reduce the tumor or result in an extended lifespan. Since I was thankfully not in that category, I began to fantasize about the possibility of forgoing treatment altogether, which quieted my sense of doom and panic.

Further research answered the questions about my emotional state. Anything I might do to assuage the stress I was experiencing after dealing with the school lawsuit could help me feel more upbeat, and could help me have a better quality of life. But I found no evidence that these psychological interventions could cure the cancer or prevent its recurrence. Wilber, in a phone call with me during this time, suggested that modalities such as guided imagery, meditation, and affirmations could indeed assist in my treatment and prevention of future recurrence along with the traditional scientific methods.

Whereas positive thinking is always welcome, there are those who understand that an inability to maintain a sunny disposition during cancer treatment might well lead to feelings of guilt within the patient and her family. This became an issue in November 2010, when my daughter informed me she was pregnant. What was I to do now? If my cancer and my fight for health caused Erica high levels of stress during her pregnancy, she might develop high blood pressure (which my mother had during her pregnancy with me) or heart disease. Further, the baby might be born premature or at a low birth weight, both of which could result in serious health problems, and in the worst-case scenario she might miscarry the baby. There was also the chance that the baby might be born with asthma and/or allergies, which run in our family and which Erica experienced throughout her life.

The alternative would be to suppress/repress those emotions and not discuss my condition with my pregnant daughter. This was my normal mode of functioning as I tried, in vain, to create a normal and happy home for my little tribe. But denying my true emotions

180

would just make me feel lonely, and would make her feel alienated from her mother. This would cause both of us more pain than sharing the unvarnished truth, I decided, and would add to my burden of feeling guilty for adding this variable to our lives. Neither positive nor negative emotions affect survival, and therefore I felt that I could share my daily thoughts and feelings with her.

There is a danger among cancer support groups and books when patients are urged to keep a consistently positive mindset. I understand cancer was not caused by my negative attitude nor was it made worse by my thoughts of being a victim or scapegoat. I read through studies that showed patients with a positive attitude lived longer, yet some critics noted the studies were based on anecdotal evidence from too small a sample and used questionable research methods.

There have been those who believed that people with certain personality types were more likely to get cancer. I had imagined that my stressful life had taught my immune system to ward off malevolent changes in my cells. At the same time I believed that neurotic people and introverts were at the highest risk of cancer. Along with that, I had read that specific personality types would affect the likelihood that a person with cancer might die. This was an area that terrified me, since I had such a negative view of who I was and what type of future I would have.

After ascertaining whether my beliefs were grounded or just part of magical or mythical thinking, I found research attempting to link personality and cancer survival was limited, poorly designed, or not very well controlled. Barbara Ehrenreich's *Bright-Sided* criticizes the tyranny of positivity within many areas, particularly within the medical establishment. She devotes an entire chapter to the misapprehension of "Smile or Die: The Bright Side of Cancer." She describes hundreds of websites, newsletters, support groups, breast cancer books from first- and third-person perspectives, and "even a glossy upper-middlebrow monthly magazine, *Mamm*" (p. 21). But Ehrenreich does a disservice to those of us who have discovered there can indeed be transformative potential in having a life-threatening disease, which will be discussed in a later chapter.

I re-read *Grace and Grit* to see if Treya concentrated on maintaining a positive attitude. Treya's lump was discovered shortly before her wedding to Wilber. As in my case, she was assured that it was probably nothing. I was repeatedly told that 80% of women with my mammogram results do not have cancer. Next I was assured that 80% of the women with no felt breast mass did not have cancer, until I was told that I had the same type of cancer as 80% of women who do have cancer. Treya's cancer, unfortunately, was a rampaging malignancy with slim hope of recovery. The appropriate attitude for Treya would have been to express whatever emotion she felt like expressing. *Grace and Grit* remains a moving and unbearably touching love story for the ages, and it ends with Treya's transformative experience confronting her own death five years later. But I am not situated anywhere near that tender, frightening, ennobling, and transformational context. As my doctor told me, "You have run-of-the-mill breast cancer." I revisit Ken and Treya's story often to glean what I can of their spiritual journey, and to understand where I am situated, personally, medically, and culturally.

The Mayo Clinic considers the demand for positive thinking as a means of curing or helping with treatment to be a cultural myth:

> **Truth:** There is no scientific proof that a positive attitude gives you an advantage in cancer treatment or improves your chance of being cured. What a positive attitude can do is improve the quality of your life during cancer treatment and beyond. You may be more likely to stay active, maintain ties to family and friends, and continue social activities. In turn, this may enhance your feeling of well-being and help you find the strength to deal with your cancer. (Mayo Clinic)

I could not bear any thought of a "tyranny of positive thinking." I would never skip and smile through a very real assault on my body, with a very real possibility that my life might end. I am now a free person who feels what I need to feel at any discrete moment, and understand that emotions dissipate as all transient states do. I did not want to remain forever vigilant in repressing these natural tides of despair/equilibrium. I didn't want to think about being at my sexiest and wearing red shoes to chemotherapy, as some books on breast cancer advise. Is it wrong to be afraid? I believed I would learn more from dealing with those states than by actively attempting to repress them.

If I could not feel free to experience my natural emotions of fear, doubt, and anxiety to my health providers, then I might be tempted to turn to ineffective methods of cancer treatment. Furthermore, I might stop following the protocols and medical advice that are crucial for my survival.

Cultural Fit and Mutual Understanding

I had a strong desire to fit into my various cultures. I longed for mutual understanding with the integral community's values and was determined to test my own values by the rightness of its collective belief system.

- Will I choose the negative victim cultural identity of my family?
- Have I committed some karmic evil against my family or others that will be paid back in suffering and death?
- Which of the beliefs found within integral spirituality fit into or with my own cobbled-together beliefs?
- Would I be better off following Jewish or Buddhist beliefs about dealing with death and/or dying?
- Will my doctor and other caregivers provide emotional support and have a positive influence on my healing?

An article in the *Annals of Behavioral Medicine* implies that physicians and caregivers at places such as Sloan-Kettering would greet me with a culture of care and concern, but with this caveat: "We urge positive psychologists to rededicate themselves to a positive psychology based on scientific evidence rather than wishful thinking" (Coyne & Tennen, 2010). This implies that although the staff would be comforting and positive, they would be positive within the boundaries of scientific evidence. They would not lie to me or sugarcoat test results.

I have already introduced my family and the culture in which I was raised. By the time of my diagnosis, I was deeply embedded in yet another culture, the integral community, and more specifically, Wilber's framing of the culture of self, community, nation, and spirit. What could I take from *Grace and Grit* and the Integral framework in general? Treya served as my role model of integral consciousness from whom I could learn, whatever the outcome of my battle. As Wilber writes in the forward to the second edition of *Grace and Grit*:

> Treya's story is every person's story. It might seem that Treya "had it all": intelligence, beauty, charm, integrity, a happy marriage, a wonderful family. But, like all of us, Treya had her own doubts, insecurities.... But Treya fought the good fight with all of those shadows...and she won, by any definition of the word "win." Treya's story speaks to all of us because she met those nightmares head on, with courage and dignity and grace....How, instead of closing down and becoming bitter and angry, she greeted the world with love in her heart. How she met cancer with "passionate equanimity." (pp. xii-xiii)

As I collapsed into terror off and on during this time, my mind spiraled back to the fatal ending of Treya's story. At home I studied the passage where Wilber explains his understanding of God, and I recognized anew that I shared that same feeling. "God," to many in the Integral spiritual community, does not connote a male or female or animal anthropomorphic figure, "but rather a pure awareness, or consciousness as such, that is *what* there is and *all* there is, a consciousness that one cultivates in meditation and actualizes in daily life. This mystical understanding was absolutely central to Treya, and to me, and to our life together" (Wilber, 1991, p. 23).

The intersection of mind, body, spirit, and cultural history is central to the theory of biocognition (Martinez, 2009). Culture impacts the triggering and activation of our genes by the impact of our culturally transmitted psychological wounds to our immune
184

systems. Biocognition posits that there are three archetypal wounds that can have this negative effect on our genes: shame, abandonment, and betrayal. When these are activated during the simultaneous course of transmitting intimacy and love, they become tightly interwoven into our body/mind.

There is an immunological response to these wounds, and upon reflection I could see clearly how the sensibilities of my nuclear family were reinforced up to and through the issues of harassment from the three men at my high school. Once again, I had no doubt as to how and why I had become ill. It goes beyond the biological fact that stress releases cortisol, which accentuates pro-inflammatory responses that can cause illnesses. It is the wound that causes the release of the cortisol, and thus the wound's effects run deep. It was my repeated psychological wounds, I realized, not just the most recent episode that led to my cancers.

With my two guides, Lorraine and Patricia, I uncovered and began healing these lifelong wounds. It was all too easy for me to intellectually report the episodes of my life that caused hurt, but when I was asked "how it *felt* to be wounded," I had great difficulty recalling.

Once I was able to feel into my body, Lorraine had me "plant seeds" inside myself in order to begin understanding that there was a rich interior life accessible to me. Whenever I spoke to either Lorraine or Patricia and could not associate a feeling with the episode being recalled, I knew we had to dig more deeply into my ability to associate feelings with the recollections. This was deep and time-consuming work for us as we explored the trauma vortex or field together.

According to biocognition, the healing field for abandonment is restored by a commitment to self. This was exceedingly difficult for me, a people-pleaser, but I found I didn't need to be aggressive with others. I just needed to stand my ground on behalf of myself. Sometimes this meant saying "no" to a family member or friend because I needed to nourish myself.

I had been shamed numerous times by my mother and her sisters, and biocognition honors the healing field for handling such an old and toxic injury. This was another major area for me to tackle since it involved setting boundaries. My personality type calls me to give unconditionally to another. To set a boundary meant that I had to say "no" or "stop" somewhere. Being betrayed by a friend or colleague led me to the healing field of loyalty to myself.

All of the woundings I described in the early chapters of this book came through my lack of caution around those with different value systems. Looking after my mother was more important than getting in touch with my own emotions or body-states. Compounding this was the fact that a vacuum of self-knowledge was reflected back to me by my Southern culture of the late 1950's and early 1960's. To resolve this deficit meant working with my current relationships. I had to conduct my intimate relationships, friendships, and acquaintances through my inner healing truths. Behaving in this manner was not meant to curry favor with others, but to set up the proper brain functioning, immunological responses, and psychological fields to further my healing processes. Given the seriousness of my illnesses, I knew only dedicated and hard work on my relationships would help me change my psychoimmunological fields.

The System or Structure

The affirmation "Don't worry, be happy. Know that God loves you" can be of great sustenance to one's interior subjective sense of well-being. But does it translate into anything objectively verifiable and replicable that can be trusted? In other words, is the mortality rate lower for people who attend religious services? Attending religious services is certainly cheaper than purchasing statin drugs, but the objective results do not offer conclusive evidence: for healthy people, attendance reduces mortality by 18%, but so does eating fruits and vegetables and having a mammography.

I began to wonder:

- How would I recreate my own ecology—my personalized post-surgical life?
- What would the economic impact of my illness be on me and my family?

- Which scientific test results showing which conclusions would I would trust and follow?
- What would being a patient at Sloan-Kettering in New York City be like?
- Should I permit my pregnant daughter to visit me and see me post-surgery, as well as others who are terribly ill?
- Would my friends and family be able to make the trip to New York to visit me, or would I be alone during my treatments?
- Would I have access to the Internet and be able to do research for my course?
- What type of patients would I be roomed with?
- Would the staff permit me to make some decisions about my care and treatment?
- What ways of communication, organizing structures, decision-making systems, conflict resolution procedures, reward/penalty systems, accountability systems, bioregions, and geopolitical locations would I be embedded in and surrounded by?

Societies are examined over time (historical) and space (geographical). I next turned to examine the functional fit of my social systems (e.g., systems theory, the ecological web of life, and environmental networks). The content of this quadrant goes from micro to macro levels of existence, from the smallest to the largest structures. The conduct of each student within my class, to all of my classes, to the entire school, to the New Jersey school system, to the United States public education system, to all students world-wide, we all fit into Russian nesting dolls of systems within systems within systems—*ad infinitum*.

Another fascinating new perspective calls for cancer to be fought on the systemic level rather than just concentrating on the individual cancer cell(s). The ecology and environment of the area where the mutated cells occur need to be addressed. Change the environment, and the cancer cells cannot survive. Certainly Patricia's cell level meditations had me concentrate at this systemic level.

There is clear interest in the paths of the interior-individual and the interior-collective in the area of cancer treatment along with the paths of the exterior-individual and the exterior-collective. For example, The American Psychosocial Oncology Society is dedicated to investigating the psychological, social, behavioral, and spiritual aspects of cancer as well as exploring innovative methods of treating the disease. At the top of their suggestions I note that they echo Wilber's dictum that "one size does not fit all" and "no two breast cancers are exactly alike." As a result, the "best" treatment plan for each woman differs. The personalized approach to breast cancer treatment involves making decisions on the basis of many factors, including the type of cancer, the stage of disease, the results of biomarker testing, the genetic make-up of the tumor, and a woman's individual preferences. The approach to lung cancer is similar and explores the individualized nature of each case.

What I could not find in the "survivor" sections of the various organizations' literature was information on spiritual issues. Psychosocial information was included in most pamphlets, however, which gave me a clearer idea of how to optimize my chances of survival. When reviewing my blog, I saw how often my moods changed, from serene to agitated, from despairing to hopeful. These moods are transient features of everyone's psyche and are difficult to pin to survival statistics. More telling are *traits*, such as extroversion; dispositional pessimism; and situational factors such as stress and social support systems.

This is the basic outline of the Integral framework, but my work in deepening my alignment with it was far from done. There are books by medical theorists and practitioners on what constitutes integrative medicine and integral health, but there was no guide for me as an integral patient. For that alignment I had to apply the deeper aspects of Integral Theory to my personal condition. I had to adapt the key tenets of Integral Medicine to the patient's perspective, and then create an understanding of what integral healing might entail. Because Integral Theory embraces body, mind, and spirit, I integrated traditional, complementary, and alternative approaches toward healing the three aspects of human life.

I noted something that Sloan-Kettering had long ago discovered. Among the women whom I mentored and interviewed for this book,

188

there seemed to be similarity in the timing for *coming to terms* with her illness. Women who brushed off their treatment as just something that had to be conquered before life could return to a normal ebb and flow seemed to hit the onset of *coming to terms* deeply and sometimes abruptly after two years. It appears that women who utilized denial understood on some profound level after two years that something unique and troubling had occurred. They could no longer include their cancer experience as part of their ordinary lives. It was at this mark when Sloan-Kettering and I saw women needing a support group to do the healing of *coming to terms* that had not been seriously addressed previously.

I am at the three-year mark after diagnosis, and although I believe I have *come to terms* with my illness, I joined a support group to do this stage of the healing process in as integral a manner as I am capable.

With the aid of this wide-ranging yet specific framework, I learned to adapt my healing to my unique life circumstances.

PART 3

ADAPTATION

CHAPTER ELEVEN

Integral Healing

My diagnoses called me to connect with the wisdom of ancient traditions as well as the knowledge of cutting-edge science. Patricia Kay and Lorraine Antine reminded me that I was not only evolving along with humanity; I had a singular and generational tie to my ancestors that could help me during my medical travails. I knew from prior experience that when I put all parts of the Integral framework into service, something radical—call it psychoactive—would happen: I would experience a profound shift in consciousness and feel as though I were "one with all of creation." This spiritual state permitted me to incorporate all meaningful healing modalities in whatever guise they might arrive, be they through prayer or visualizations, chemotherapy or massage.

By now it should be evident that healing is not just a property of the physical body (Upper Right); there is a corresponding emotional/psychological body in the "I" quadrant that must be healed (Upper Left), a cultural belief that needs clarification (Lower Left), and a system-wide view of medical protocols that impact healing as well (Lower Right). I once again went to the dictionary to assist me in understanding the tetra-arising concept of healing. The Merriam-Webster Dictionary offers the following definition of healing:

1. To make sound or whole
2. To restore to health
3. To cause (an undesirable condition) to be overcome
4. To restore to original purity or integrity
5. To return to a sound state

The Free Dictionary adds a spiritual component to the term: To restore (a person) to spiritual wholeness.

The Key Tenets of Integral Healing

I was focused on my personal healing and did not dwell on the perspectives of the medical professionals treating me. Their perspectives would be different, of course, although I considered possible common themes. Dr. Marilyn Schlitz has summarized the tenets of Integral Medicine, and I translated her perspectives to that of the patient as experienced during my personal journey:

1. Integral healing is a dynamic, holistic, life-long process that exists to widen and deepen relationships with self, culture, and nature.

Although it is clear from its definition that healing can be used broadly, it most often refers to healing of the physical body, as in the healing of a disease, illness, or injury. The word is also frequently used to indicate healing of mental, psychological, or emotional conditions. For those who are spiritually inclined, "to make sound or whole" would have to include the spiritual dimension of life as well. Not explicitly present is Wilber's consideration of "sickness," which envelops illness within a cultural construct.

From an integral perspective, health indicates preservation of all the preconditions for developing and maintaining systems that permit: flexibility of coping mechanisms; positive adaptive responses; and transcendence of self. Transcendence is part of our experience of the world. Here, transcendence means stepping outside of the personal egoic perspective and seeing the world from a universal perspective.

In selecting Sloan-Kettering as my treating hospital I understood the physicians would be treating my body, the external objective part of me with scientifically established medical protocols. But I was just as concerned with supporting my self with meditation, guided imagery, and affirmations. I wondered at the time whether the doctors would encourage me to join a cancer support group that would satisfy my longing for collective support.

Each quadrant is tied to the other three. An emotional state, such as my fear of chemo, has a corresponding brain state in the physical organism of my body. Sloan-Kettering has medical protocols that directed me to seek specific treatment for the best statistical outcome, but my fear of the treatment made me more liable to join a support group.

By widening my relationship with my self, my culture, and the planet, I was stretching myself toward advanced states of commitment and principled behavior. Once I committed myself to living a life guided by spiritual principles within the Integral framework, I felt the utmost humility and fundamental awe of all the forces of creation. I could no longer exclude consideration of unpleasant elements within my life, at whatever distance I might initially place them. Contracting cancer is terribly unfair at any stage of life, but seeing the disease as part of my overall destiny and incorporating it into my personal spiritual quest was a helpful coping strategy. It also permitted the internal coherence I sought my entire life.

Narrative medicine and writing for healing gave me the courage to begin writing from my emotional depths about my experiences. As I wrote, I witnessed changes in my understanding of my life events. Some traumatic experiences became muted through seeing how they led me toward greater empathy. Other disappointments could be placed in the context of "stuff happens." I was no longer the victim; I was the Narrator of my own life, and I reclaimed the right to understand it from my perspective.

I acknowledge that my approach to relationships, themes, and events in my life may be unique. This approach is based on a singular lens that changed over the years— an evolutionary process to which I opened up. The victimhood I felt after my cancer diagnosis would eventually segue into appreciation for the insights yielded by the pain and fear. Painful emotions morphed into the awe and humility of which I have spoken. I am still learning to trust that process.

By deepening my relationships, I chose to reject rigidness and to attune myself to my open heart. Instead of contracting back when I felt attacked, I could move forward in curiosity about what was happening. My connection with the Ground of Being permits me to act with as much truth as I am capable, and to act with as much inclusive love as possible. That is the ground of my healing process, the bonding of the four quadrants.

2. Integral healing is about transformation, growth, and the restoration of wholeness.

Transformation is a term adopted by many spiritual and religious adherents to a process that is more easily explained by the synonym "metamorphosis," which is defined by the Merriam Webster Dictionary as a change of physical form, structure, or substance especially by supernatural means, or a striking alteration in appearance, character, or circumstances. Some schools consider the concept that a supernatural entity causes or assists during transformation, but my understanding of supernatural is more in line with the concept of "trans-rational" (i.e., beyond rational understanding). There is an active component to all of these terms and I prefer to see them as organic and process-oriented.

My health is a process in which I develop a progressively inclusive meaning-making system that allows me to function, to heal, and to grow in the face of present and future changes, challenges, and the ultimate end of earthly existence. Regardless of what changes— myself, my body, my relationships, and the world in which I exist—I will continue to evolve and my essential self will effectuate similar changes in others. Transformation implies a fundamental shift toward greater inclusiveness of understanding and awareness, and toward greater joy and love.

Moving away from the idea of the atomistic individual self into self-transcendence, I had previously experienced transcendent awareness of something that appeared just out of sight. Pain, hopelessness, or relief seemed to trigger access to these peak experiences, which researcher Elliott Dacher cheekily refers to as "peek experiences" (2011, p. 8). Holding onto these insights is another matter, and living from such high places is a holy venture. The ability to access and sustain higher levels of awareness requires a leap of consciousness, a move to self-transformation instead of self-regulation or self-improvement (Ibid, p. 13). These transcendent moments of pure Spirit with bliss as the constituent context are

194

slippery topics. One definition of self-transcendence states it is an act or condition of going/being beyond ego, usually as the result of love, service, non-egoic discipline, or undivided attention for another. This technique is considered essential for spiritual and psychological progress, and it is also a state or condition in which spiritual ecstasy is experienced.

One trick employed by the ego is to flatter itself into believing that puffing itself up equals transcendence. I've witnessed battles among people who claim their egos are smaller than another person's. There is a corollary to this concern: spiritual bypassing. It is not unusual to meet spiritual seekers who have suppressed or denied their emotions in order to simulate an experience of wholeness, which is precisely the opposite of what is intended by transformation.

A second concern is the contrast between many spiritual practitioners' understanding of transformation with the Integral model's conception of it. Rather than advocate for me to go to a cave to meditate until I am transformed by my illness, I understand Integral Psychology to encourage engagement with the world (Shirazi, as cited in Schlitz, p. 240). It also urges me to incorporate both paths of spiritual seekers: the evolutionary and the involutionary. These terms represent the tendency of religion or spiritual teachings to focus on one aspect of growth and ignore the other, rather than embrace them both. Evolutionary or ascending practices teach the ever-seeking attainment of perfection, into Christ-consciousness, for example. Descending traditions seek perfection from the higher energy of the Divine and grounding of the individual in their earthly lives through such concepts as grace.

3. My conscious awareness of who and what I am, where I exist, my various perspectives, emotions, behaviors and worldviews, will shape and has shaped my attitude toward the cancers and infection I experienced.

My body, my mind, and my spirit all interact in shaping how I evolved and developed over the course of my illness, and continue to change and transform my relationships and me. My heart has broken open with endless love many times since I was diagnosed, and this breaking open will continue into the future. As my understanding develops into more comprehensive waves, I have questions about the doctor's medical chart:

In today's complex universe, is it fair to ask where do we as a culture locate illness? If I am located in a sickly biosphere, was I ever healthy?

Since I am a "holon," an entity that truly cannot be separated from the entirety, to whom do I go to be healed? (Dacher, as cited in Schlitz, p. 8)

And where does healing come from? Where do we situate well-being and peace of mind?

I returned home after the lung cancer surgery to find the radon content of my home registered a score of 4.4, the equivalent of me having smoked eight cigarettes a day for the 37 years I lived there. My lung cancer could have originated from a naturally occurring gas seeping through the base of my house.

My meaning-making system seized on the cancer as originating from external sources. If I could just pin the cause of my illnesses on radon, harassment, or random mutating cells, then perhaps I bore no role in becoming ill. This perspective also strengthened my attachment to a biomedical awareness of my illnesses.

Realizing that I am far more than just my body or an illness within my body, however, I was able to search for a transcendent quality to my situation. I was fixated on the elimination of cancer from my body, but to achieve true healing I had to look beyond a narrow search for pleasure and the avoidance of pain. This pleasure/pain principle is known in both spiritual and psychological realms. It might sound counterintuitive, but without a transcendent understanding of healing, we embrace a perpetual cycle of hope and fear. Here I sit, "cancer-free" they tell me, and I fear every semi-annual cancer scan. What if it has come back? How do I hold onto my status of being "cancer-free"?

Friends have reported vomiting or having panic attacks the day before their routine scans. Although some report launching their lives onto new and exciting paths, others become so fearful of the cancer returning they refuse to rock the boat. They never truly get on with their lives for fear the next scan will plunge them back into medical purgatory. Stability might be attained, but life falls into a dull, fear-based pattern.

Finding healing "out there" energized me at first. I became obsessed with institutions and protocols. I feared pain and wanted to be assured that I would feel none or only a trifle during treatments. But when I embraced an integral understanding that there is nothing "outside" of me, I was called back in a profound manner to reconnect and ground myself. Blame of an external "other" reinforced the old "us versus them" dualism of my family and my culture. I realized I would have to let hope and fear go, down to my core, although I have retained them in the telling of my story. It would overwhelm people who ask about my complicated medical rollercoaster if I were to insert transcendent beliefs into the narrative. As for the men at my school who caused me so much psychic and physical suffering, I let go, but I have not forgotten. When the memories cause me pain, I let go of them as well.

4. Using an integral perspective on my complex situation requires I deeply examine my core assumptions of reality.

Integral Theory requires me to disperse my healing attention to four realms: physical health and illness require healing; emotional health and sickness require healing; mental health and sickness require healing; and spiritual health and sickness require healing.

I had not considered complementary and alternative medical approaches to cancer at first; it took coming to terms with what I faced to bring these modalities into my conscious awareness. Both Patricia and Lorraine shared their expertise in directing me to homeopathic and integrative practices and remedies. I trusted them both and thus overcame my skepticism of some of the suggested cancer-attacking methods.

I cried over a blog entry written by a 40-year-old woman with aggressive cancer who refused conventional treatment in lieu of an unproven protocol offered by an online company. For weeks she gushed about how she was beating the conventional medical world of pain and surgery. Then the entries ended, and her husband posted that she had passed away. This did not prove that only conventional treatment saves lives, but it did alert me to the propensity of fear to drive us away from combining alternative and complementary modalities with conventional means of fighting this multifactorial illness.

Prayer, meditation, and visualization marry modern medicine in my approach to healing. I had read enough studies to know that even conventional medicine has recognized their effectiveness. These techniques serve as "a bridge, connecting the conscious or unconscious, physiological or psychological activities, or experiences" (Schlitz, as cited in Schlitz, p. 229). These techniques bridge my concept of who was being healed and by what: I was participating in my own healing in a way that re-energized long-held wisdom and cutting-edge science. Larry Dossey considers this the "respiritualization of medicine" (Dossey, as cited in Schlitz, p. 321), and believes that medicine will either be respiritualized or it will cease being a comprehensive profession.

5. We are at a watershed of human evolution where we have developed an understanding of all of the world's knowledge as well as an unparalleled understanding of our own consciousness.

"[T]he scientific quest is incomplete without data from many domains of inquiry, and without various kinds of knowing...." (Schlitz, p. xxxviii). Holding the wisdom offered by major integral thinkers, I was called to incorporate scientific, sensory-based, logical, self-analytical, integrative, nondual traditions, and evolutionary consciousness. As long as the four quadrants were honored, the Integral framework permitted me to embrace that which resonated most.

After years of dealing with chronic stress, and the times when fight-or-flight ruled my behavior, I worried I had a diminished ability to cope with my new health crises. Yet as I held this fear, I also realized I had a limitless—and untouched—reservoir of support: my state of consciousness. This determined the lens through which I

198

perceived the reality I was living within, and this lens determines the kind of thoughts my brain produces and the patterns of my moods. It determines the extent of my vulnerability to others, which I admit to feeling.

It also determines the extent of my creative powers. With a narrow lens through which to see myself and my world, the less capable I was of demonstrating creativity. For example, my mother never encouraged me or gave me support to explore my own creative ability to write poetry, an area where she wanted to keep her genius paramount. It has only been recently, with the writing of this book and the enlarged lens by which I see myself that I have begun to write poetry.

I realized with great relief that I could situate my healing potential from within the expansiveness of my own consciousness. This spaciousness goes down to the spaces between each molecule of my body. When I am in pain, that is all I can think of; but when I do as both Lorraine and Patricia suggested, which is create a space around the pain that is not pain, I can turn this subject of my awareness into an object of my awareness, making it only part of what I can be aware of. It no longer overwhelms me; I can imagine Spirit/the Divine/God breathing into that space, opening up my heart to the wisdom of what I really am.

This expansiveness is identical to the evolutionary experience, or "moving forward" in the creative sense. The evolutionary direction of reality provided me with a meaningful, empowering, and inspiring creation myth. I came to view all life as being in a mutually enriching relationship, with the scientific and religious domains inseparable from one another.

I took to heart that I could actively participate in the evolution of consciousness—for myself, for others, and for our systems. My participation had to be with the Divine, Spirit, God or the Ground of Being, and our co-creation followed the deepest patterns of nature and the entirety of the universe. But I could not do this critical work from a sense of egoic self-importance. I couldn't make hubris the soil into which I planted my healing; it would not take root. I couldn't play integral healing like a puzzle where I put a quadrant here, a state of consciousness there, and a physical practice elsewhere.

I believed the Integral framework could move my healing forward. Did this mean I could become cancer-free by using integral principles? Yes and no. Of course I wanted to be free of cancer and move forward with my life, and took steps to passionately engage an integral healing methodology.

At the same time I embraced the "not-knowing" of what I was doing and the uncertainty of the results. I was deeply curious about what would happen with my health. It might mean the quiet and beautiful acceptance of my own death, or it might mean living each day with profound humility and awe.

I wanted to align my consciousness with all that was yet unborn, impossible to know with and by ego, and inherently liberated from time and space. I had learned to be at that sweet spot between moving forward with a health-affirming program and remaining curious from a neutral consciousness about what might manifest.

My healing journey also made me curious about what Wilber called the "marriage of sense and soul," which is also the title of his 1998 book. I was joined with sisters and brothers across the centuries and the continents in exploring this aspect of evolutionary culture. The developmental attention the Integral model pays to body, mind, and spirit in self, culture, and planet made me appreciate it was not just my personal healing at stake. I became acutely aware that my personal relationships needed healing, as did my culture and the planet. This all-level healing awareness felt precisely right to me— not off-topic or a distraction. I looked back over my attempts to heal various relationships. I lost one friendship during the acute stage of my illness after becoming entangled in a contest over who had the saddest life. Only during the dissolution of this long relationship did I come to confront my repetition of victimhood, and I realized the friendship was best laid to rest.

"Unconditional love" is a phrase often associated with parenting. My error had been a failure to create the same safety for me that I attempted to provide for my child. Such love is not what is intended by the spiritual traditions. We do not shower our children with unconditional love by approving every one of their misdeeds. Rather, we love them by guiding them, by regulating their behavior with rules, and by protecting our boundaries so that we are not harmed by errant choices. One young mother I know of actually permitted her four-year-old daughter to hit her and kick the father in the crotch, all in the name of unconditional love.

The need to heal our culture also became a critical issue for me, and remains so. "Healing the planet" might sound as vacuous as a pageant contestant's hope for world peace, but spiritual practices tell us that by our own awakening we do indeed heal the planet. By devoting the proper alignment of my healing energy to myself and my relationships, I was creating a resonant frequency with my loved ones and anyone with whom I interacted. Incorporating appropriate boundaries for my well-being and healthy functioning while permitting spiritually healthy openness is referred to as chesed, agape, bhakti, or metta. Practicing these ancient directions not only led to my awakening, but it touched on the reality that the state of my mind was a reflection of the state of all minds. I truly believed the spiritual practices I adopted created a benefit for all.

6. The aim of integral healing is an expanded consciousness that embraces and includes wholeness, peace, love, and joy, where wisdom binds the Left- and Right-Hand paths.

The aim of integral healing is to utilize as complete and as comprehensive an approach as possible when facing ill health, while remaining constrained by the pragmatic realities of time, insurance limitations, and the physical dynamics of the illness. As complementary and alternative modalities become more accepted, integral healing embraces a larger world that includes, yet is not limited to, the physical, spiritual, psychological, and cultural manifestations of illness. A comprehensive definition of wholeness is useful, but its application must be applied to the granular life of the individual.

Wilber once referred to consciousness by the metaphor of a spectrum, which can be defined as a range of values of a quantity or set of related quantities. It is also a broad sequence or range of related qualities, ideas, or activities. Since being in a spectrum implies relatedness, I presumed a change, disturbance, or development in any part of the spectrum was bound to affect my other bandwidths

(Shirazi, as cited in Schlitz, pp. 238-239). My illness and its cultural context initially created massive disruptions within my consciousness. I first plunged deeper into feeling like a victim and made decisions based on fear, so it was obvious to me that I could correct this imbalance by working to strengthen my positive values and mindsets without the aid of magical thinking.

I tried my normal meditation technique only to discover that it no longer brought me to expanded consciousness. I felt no peace, joy, or love. In fact, I felt disappointment that during this trying time my practice was failing me. I received no joy from my normal creative endeavors. I stopped cooking since my senses of smell and taste had become distorted and unreliable. My bones hurt when I underwent chemo, and my chest stung with sharp stabs from the nerve damage I suffered after having my ribs spread during surgery. Even my hair hurt as it began to fall out. Rather than turn into a hopelessly mutilated creature, I sought instead to find other avenues within the totality of reaching expanded consciousness that represents human potential. One avenue I did not choose was the intake or ingestion of exogenous substances. I figured that I was on enough strong drugs, and self-medicating might skew my internal balance to the point where the prescribed medications would not be effective.

I switched to chanting, for singing had always been an avenue of exhilaration and creative expression for me. I found poetry, art, and spiritual works I'd never explored, and visualizations that reinvigorated my capacity to participate in my healing. I also explored areas that scientist, religious scholar, and Jewish author Jeff Levin proposed. What might happen to ideas about healing if we came to accept that love is a health-promoting agent, as Levin suggests (Schlitz, p. 231)? What if love is not the end product of being healed, but an actual healing modality? Levin explored this possibility, which I found foundational for my healing. The caveat is that each personality type filters the definition through a different lens, and my filter had to be adjusted before I could use the love-as-gift to others as a healing agent. My deep-rooted belief that perhaps I did not warrant love prevented me from initially embracing this approach. A new lightning strike would cause me to tumble back into victimhood, closing my positive emotional stance and effectively preventing the rooting of love within me. Culturally, however, I did accept that love
202

is permissible for those who are quite ill. I opened myself as much as possible to love from my family, friends, and spiritual caregivers, Patricia and Lorraine. Their ability to transmit love was infectious.

My dog Chloe was one agent of love that I had no problem staying open for. During the treatment sessions I attended with other cancer patients I heard stories of their special relationship with their pets. Several reported their previously healthy pets, usually cats, were diagnosed with similar cancers. Judith Orloff, M.D., agrees:

> Could it be possible for one life to so empathize with another that it can sense, even assume illness? Certainly, something to contemplate. As a physician I know that love can create miracles that defy logical explanation. Selfless giving resonates with such mystery. How wondrous and far reaching compassion can be among all living beings. Each of us is capable of limitless love. The monumental implications of this fact continue to reveal themselves over the years, always giving me chills and re-clarifying my emotional priorities. (Orloff, 2011)

What if the forgiveness of all my tormentors added to my healing potential, as implied by the Stanford Forgiveness Projects (Harris et al., 2006)? Published in 2001, the project studied a "forgiveness intervention" with a cohort of victimized or aggrieved participants. Participants were schooled in taking less personal offense, blaming the offender less, and offering more personal and situational understanding of the offender and of oneself. Results indicated the possibility that skills-based forgiveness training may prove effective in reducing anger as a coping style, reducing perceived stress and physical health symptoms, and thereby helping to reduce the effect of stress on immune and cardiovascular functioning. I might have perceived this practice as a guilt-inducing religious mandate to forgive those who had hurt me. But when I engaged it sincerely and deeply, forgiveness was validated as a tetra-arising, interwoven element to continue expanding my consciousness.

From this practice came the understanding that I would have to offer forgiveness to all the grievances of the past and present.

Even if the agent of my mistreatment proved unable to meet me for reconciliation, as had been true within my husband's family, I still could create peace of mind by no longer obsessing over the hurts. I came to deeply understand why the fourth stage of healing, appreciation, could include the gift of the illness itself. Nothing urged me to deal with my pattern of victimization more than this profound crisis, and nothing provided a better vehicle than the Integral framework.

With these six tenets revised to apply to the patient and not the practitioner, I had the framework by which to apply the integral toolkit to my own healing.

From Diagnosis to Healing

Let's see what happens when we place the term diagnosis within the Integral model. I knew "something wasn't right" within my body once I received the problematic mammogram. In alignment with my cultural beliefs, I sought out medical experts to see what symptoms emerged, and how my culture and the prevailing wisdom categorized the malady. Every disease can be explored by this type of quadrant analysis, which is the primary reason I adopted a full-quadrant approach to what turned out to be three serious surgeries and a healing phenomenon.

In *Health and Healing*, Andrew Weil discusses alternative healing methods that are more apt to appeal to certain cultural demographics. In my area of New Jersey, there would be little support for seeking out most complementary and alternative remedies, whereas the San Francisco Bay area would be far more receptive. I was willing to embrace some alternative methods in addition to traditional scientific remedies, and to wrap them around my spiritual practice. With guidance, I adopted an alternative approach of using herbs; homeopathic remedies that did not interfere with my chemotherapy; radiant heating from an amethyst crystal mattress; cell level meditation; and food as medicine. I deepened my practice of integral spirituality because surrounding all of the quadrants and at their base is Spirit, the Ground of All Being, or the Ultimate.

I realized there was a polarity between being cured of cancer and being restored to health.

What is being healed?
How will healing occur?
Who will be involved in the healing process?

Integral Theory directs us to a possible approach to these questions, but it is a complex approach to truly complex questions. Both illness and healing can originate on separate planes of understanding. The basic structure of existence of which we are all aware is the physical, wherein an "I" exists. Cancer is a confounding disease that originates with one cell that begins to endlessly replicate, but what causes that growth? Is it simply bad luck, genetics, geography, or a soup of unknown catalysts?

Body, Mind and Spiritual Healing

The quadrants address body, matter, and mind. I took this a step up from the physical, and considered the spiritual aspects of healing:

> The cure of the part should not be attempted without treatment of the whole. No attempt should be made to cure the body without the soul. Let no one persuade you to cure the head until he has first given you his soul to be cured, for this is the great error of our day, that physicians first separate the soul from the body.
> – Plato

The healing of the whole calls us to the AQAL model, for with it we are assured of a treatment that embraces as many aspects of being as possible.

Within the field of my emotions and thoughts, I experienced harassment, along with its terror and stress, over a two-year period. Did that cause the mutation that caused my cancer? Did I manifest too much of a victim personality that I in some manner permitted the causal gene to mutate? Spiritually, how am I creating an open area within me for the best and most nourishing medical, social, personal, and physical systems to lead me to total healing?

When I am fully present in my body, what wisdom emerges that might integrate my thoughts and emotions?

How am I able to transform my mind from victim to co-healer?

Finally, am I able to touch the source of reality as spirit, or am I limited in my embodied consciousness?

When it comes to my physical body, I tend to engage in behaviors that lead to pleasure and avoid pain. Perhaps I had not eaten the right foods or exercised enough. Did I put non-organic and potentially dangerous compounds into my body by not washing my fruits or vegetables? Was my body so unhealthy that it permitted the cancer cells to wildly divide?

During diagnosis and until I pass away, how will I manage the energy of my body, physically, psychically, and spiritually? Have I integrated all of them as best I can, and am I endeavoring to increase the ability to manage all three?

With my mind, am I continuing to read and to self-inquire and then move to translate the theory I have incorporated into practice, or am I not making that move which is not within my comfort zone?

Spiritually, am I cultivating skillful means to move beyond my comfort zone and surrender to the Divine/Spirit/God?

Was my family's belief system about the "curse of bad luck" something I carried inside me, thus activating a self-fulfilling prophecy from the Lower-Left quadrant?

Within my body, am I working to increase my intuition in assessing others and the traps from my history?

Can I engage with new mental awareness that others might treat me differently since I became ill with not one but two cancers? Am I developed in my ability to take multiple perspectives that I will be compassionate for others who hold attitudes that might cause me to feel hurt?

Spiritually, can I hold compassion for these perspectives while championing my own needs during this trying time? Do I understand the intention that is necessary to open up to love and wisdom?

Can my attachment to the healing institutions and protocols of the Lower-Right quadrant survive critical assessments?

I want a functional fit between the treatments and the staff who administer them. I will not comply with treatment programs that violate important understandings of my body with its competencies and limitations. My medical team must be supportive, or at the very least not antagonistic, toward my desire to incorporate alternative medicine approaches in my treatment.

I want to have an open dialogue with my treatment staff and I wish to be respected for the research and understandings that I have accrued through my mental abilities.

Spiritually, how am I creating an open area within me for the best and most nourishing medical, social, personal, and physical systems to lead me to total healing?

Below I address how the other elements of the AQAL model—levels, lines, states, and types—impact health and healing. Each section deserves a book of its own, but for the sake of brevity, I have given a brief explanation here, and have expanded the elements on my web site, www.integralhealing.com.

Levels

The following is a linear trajectory of stages for integral healing that I created for my individualized treatment plan, which I have deemed an Integral Healing program:

1. Analyze the cancer diagnosis via all four quadrants.
2. Identify the cycles of healing as lightning strikes, coming to terms, adaptation, and appreciation.
3. Identify myself as co-healer, rather than a victim or even merely a patient.
4. Apply the complete Integral map to my unique situation, which means quadrants, levels, lines, states, types, and shadow.
5. Identify and contact a community of healers to assist me in my treatment journey.
6. Establish relationships with the support team I have identified.
7. Receive prescriptions/advice from healers, myself, and my support team.
8. Create a beautiful and functional setting for integral healing to take place.

I considered these eight steps as unfolding in cyclical phases with the successful completion of the first step necessary to address the second step, and so forth. My challenge was to apply as much conscious awareness to each stage so I might move on to the next level of complexity and toward a better ecology within which to heal.

Lines

Developmental lines can be assessed by observing specific behaviors and proclivities as well as testing our multiple intelligences, as developed by psychologist Howard Gardner. We each excel in some areas and do not excel in others. Perhaps we ignore these imbalances unless one line becomes critical to our livelihood or adaptive responses to a crisis.

Assessing my individual lines of development helped me create the best chance of a healthy adaptive response when I needed to be at my strongest in particular areas. The list below encompasses some of the traditionally considered multiple intelligences and names the scholar most identified with the study of that line. In dealing with healing, I benefitted from understanding my unique developmental trajectory in each line, and structured the creation of a personalized healing practice. Each line of development can be simplified by considering its core question at a particular stage in my life, as seen in the chart below:

LINE	LIFE'S QUESTION	RESEARCHER
Cognitive	*What am I aware of?*	Piaget, Kegan
Interpersonal	*How should we interact?*	Selman, Perry
Kinesthetic	*How should I physically do this?*	Gardner
Self	*Who am I?*	Loevinger
Needs	*What do I need?*	Maslow
Values	*What is significant to me?*	Graves
Moral	*What should I do?*	Kohlberg
Emotional	*How do I feel about this?*	Goleman
Spiritual	*What is of ultimate concern?*	Fowler

Table 1. Lines of development and representative researchers.

Cognitive: The cognitive line of development is concerned with how we learn things through conceptual thought, and how we grow and change in certain types of mental processes. It is related to IQ. Wilber calls this line "necessary but not sufficient" for the attainment of enlightenment, and it remains the king of them all. Cancer led me to a prolonged period of in-depth research into many topics way beyond my normal areas of concern, and this actually strengthened the development of my mental processes.

Interpersonal: How should I interact with others? How do we react to others and are we aware of their feelings? I am a good patient, comply with directions from medical staff, am easy-going, and have a high tolerance for pain. I didn't need improvement in this area.

Kinesthetic: How should I physically move and handle tasks associated with my treatment? I am not highly developed here at all, which directed me to do body work and join a gym. Physical activity lessens depression and anxiety, heightens mobility, and improves concentration.

Self: Who am I? Am I self-aware of my behavior and what my various cultural interactions deem to be acceptable? After having taken a variety of assessments over a decade, I have shown a high ego development line. Even so, it did not keep me from being psychologically injured. But blogging since 2010 and writing this book led me to deep inquiry as to who I was, and how I saw myself healing.

Needs: What do I need? Abraham Maslow wrote about the hierarchy of needs, and if anything can plunge a high-performing person down to the base of his pyramid, it is cancer. I did identify initially as a cancer victim, and I was partially sacrificed on the altar of the operating table three times in three months. I had food, water, and shelter, but for a long time I did not have assurance of continued survival.

Values: What is significant to me? This line is closely related to the "needs" category. What do I value and how has that changed since my journey with cancer? My spiritual values tended to predominate during this time as a means of great support. I wanted to share the feeling that we are all one.

Moral: I reflected on the "legacy" I might leave behind. Whose needs should I tend to first—mine? my adult students? my family?

Emotional: How do I feel about this? My emotions fluctuated wildly from one doctor visit to the next, from one diagnosis to another. I had a changing narrative as to why I had the two cancers; whether the narrative was correct or not, it permitted me to avoid feeling guilty about my role in becoming ill.

Spiritual: What is my ultimate concern? This topic looks markedly different to people at different stages of spiritual development. Cross-spiritual paths look similar at similar stages of spiritual development, whereas people can vary wildly developmentally from within one faith path.

I have analyzed and plotted my lines of development on what is called an integral psychograph (i.e., a bar chart that depicts each line of development in relation to the others). Being aware of my lines and the levels of accomplishment in each directed me to where I needed to direct more energy.

States

The term "consciousness" requires several books to explore and explain. From Wilber's perspective, the more complex the organism, the deeper, wider, and more sophisticated perspectives the entity can create. We humans are capable of the higher levels, which have no boundaries, nor do they have beginnings or ends.

What makes this subject confusing is figuring out the difference between *states* of consciousness and *stages* of consciousness. Temporary states of consciousness can become permanent traits, or stages, of consciousness. The wisdom traditions recognize three major states of consciousness: waking, dreaming, and deep formless sleep, which are temporary, and cycle throughout our life. At the same time, they correspond to three realms or worlds of being: waking brings about a gross realm of existence to our consciousness; dreaming brings about the subtle realm of consciousness; and deep formless sleep brings about access to the causal realm.

Being awake, in a dream state, or in deep formless sleep permits us to "see," or to have access to, a different realm. The fascinating human experiment is to access these non-gross states while awake and aware, which can be accomplished through state training such as meditation. I have not actually flown like a bird and felt the wind rush against my skin, as I conceived during one dream. With meditation and other forms of spiritual practice, I can access the realms of the subtle and the causal while awake and aware. Through them, wisdom and clarity arrive.

The causal state of deep formless sleep is akin to the realm I inhabited during my spiritual awakening experience at Sloan-Kettering. I could not "see" or recognize an "other" when I was in this space, since my Self and anything manifesting outside my Self was none other than me as well. I capitalize the word "Self" as a way to differentiate the felt-sense that I had from all other times that I interact with the gross realm, a small "me" that is just one of several billion on this planet. The concepts of time and space disappeared and were replaced with a difficult-to-describe sense of "being-ness," or "I-am-ness."

States can be ordinary, terrifying or blissful, and still others are extraordinary. Given that cancer has become such a powerful force in my life, I cycled through all of these varieties, including some powerful awakening and bliss-filled states. My blog, "Integral Experiences With Breast Cancer," recounts my cycling through all manner of transient states, some so powerful and novel that I had to consult books to assist me in identifying them.

State training is a significant practice for cancer patients. In time, the bliss-filled causal realm can be molded into a stage of consciousness that can be permanently accessed. Pain can be ameliorated, fear can be handled, and the "unknowability" of one's disease process can be blended into the simple in-and-out of breath. I utilized cell-level meditation and other varieties of state training during these two years to cope with whatever emotional or physical burden I was facing at that moment.

Types

The Enneagram

The Enneagram is a model of human personality that has

an uncertain origin. This personality typology reflects nine interconnected classic types of functioning, but one of the nine appears to predominate with a drive toward rectifying a core wound or fear. I have found it helpful to hold the Enneagram with the respect of a mirror that can identify parts of my personality that require further examination and development.

Once a cancer patient determines his "Enneatype," each of which emphasizes different ways of coping with illness, he can better determine his treatment plan. Don Riso and Russ Hudson's *The Wisdom of the Enneagram* and other books on the subject list the types and their overarching action principles.

These are fascinating elements for a game or an afternoon's reading, but with a serious disease the typology has more significant consequences. My first words to my doctor upon hearing that I probably had breast cancer were concerns over the people who signed up for my course. I am an Enneatype Two, the Altruist, the Caretaker, the Pleaser, the Enabler, or the Special Friend. Although I hold all typologies lightly, my typology did help me explain my primary concern. Had I been stronger in my acknowledging my needs, I would have insisted in postponing or cancelling the class, regardless of the opposition by the person in charge. There is a section in Riso and Hudson's book dealing with health and "suffering" that hit me hard: "[B]eing ill is often the only way they [Twos] can get a vacation from their responsibilities and from the demands of their superegos." (p. 143) Their guidance for me was also on-point, and became part of my healing program:

> We cannot will ourselves to love ourselves or to love others. All we can do, paradoxically, is to recognize the presence of love in ourselves and others..[O]ur essential nature is an outpouring of love—the only problem is that it is blocked by the habits and false beliefs of our personality. What is in our power is to become aware of those blockages so that our essentially loving nature can once again make itself felt and have a healing effect in our lives....It is full of joy because nothing can disappoint or frustrate it. Real love in action is unstoppable. (Riso & Hudson,

p. 149)

Sandra Maitri's book *The Spiritual Dimension of the Enneagram* includes an exploration of spirituality within each type. Her challenge rang forth to me:

> We may not experience ourselves as an indivisible part of Being, and so may not perceive that everything that occurs within our psyches and within our lives is part of the will of Being, but that does not change the fundamental truth. All it means is that our perception is filtered through the separatist lens of the personality, and so our vision is cloudy and we are not seeing reality clearly. (Maitri, p. 157)

I tried to embrace this sentiment from the heart level and not just from my intellect. When I was able to embrace and integrate the concept into my way of being, I could jettison the victim part of me. It propelled me to use illness and other physical and psychic hardships as gifts, as holy challenges to transcend the ordinary and long-held sense of being an "I" acted upon by an "other."

Archetypes

There are many ways of assessing and evaluating types: the Myers-Briggs, the Big Five, and Archetypes. In *Restoring My Soul: Finding and Living the Authentic Self*, Andrea Mathews investigates archetypes that were externalized during trauma, an experience I have had. Why do we put on masks and appropriate a false identity?

> We ask the world, without knowing we are asking, who it would like for us to be. And then we become that. Why would we do this? Because our survival is at stake. For some it is literal survival… We put on a costume and a mask and we wear it all day every day. (Mathews, p. 8)

Gayle Sulik's *Pink Ribbon Blues* tells many stories of the great wit and extroversion associated with these archetypes. Her classification of archetypes fit into my battles with cancer, my own one called the

Scapegoat with its Priest variant.

Shadow

Psychology students and integral practitioners will be aware of the term shadow, which speaks of the dark side of our psyches. Depth psychology was the means by which I chose to work through my shadow's worst emanations and liberate myself from my worst tendencies.

The shadow comprises all of our blind spots as well as the repeated errors around repressed and disowned aspects of our selves. My shadow areas involved the residual effects of past traumas that stifled my capacity to deal with ordinary interpersonal stressors. The school episode was far worse than an "ordinary interpersonal stressor," however, and therefore I place it in a special category as a dangerous, carcinogenic-encouraging stressor.

How was I to deal with my lifelong belief in being a victim/scapegoat? Victim mentality was lodged in my belief that I was helpless, my belief that my circumstances were beyond my control. Too often during my life I kept score of why bad things happened to me, and certainly my struggles with two different cancers could have triggered a crippling "Why me?" mentality. The fact that the cancers were detected after the most stressful episode of my life could have cemented this victim mentality permanently.

The school harassment situation was difficult. The men who aligned against me were the top-down administrative group in a tiny one school district where I felt powerless to challenge them. But it was my choice not to abandon my student-centric integral educational methods, and therefore I had to confront the consequences of my behavior. I had to accept responsibility for being the "righteous rebel" and all that it wrought. My ego, my self-sense, my feelings about my competency as a teacher were undermined during that time. Given my background and the serious scapegoating I endured, I naturally fell into a victim mentality—a situation I had to confront head-on at long last.

With the help of the Integral model, I was able to put myself into the minds and personalities of my foes: they saw me not as the noble teacher attempting to raise the consciousness and moral functioning of each student, but as some rebellious employee who refused to follow their direct orders to speak from a script that included no creative exercises.

I began to see myself not as a hapless victim, but as a brave warrior who had done battle and in many ways was victorious. The men could not vanquish me unless I accepted their perspective. The rest of the faculty chose to support me, and a collective belief emerged that I was not treated fairly even with the mistakes I had made. I began to shift my identity from "victim" to "co-creator" of my destiny. With that turn, the nightmares were replaced by pleseant and satisfying dreams.

Although I have attributed some responsibility for my cancer to the stress at my school, I am well aware the disease could have been triggered by factors well beyond the stress I endured. My research has shown a very strong correlation between workplace stress and cancer, but if my body responded to severe stress, then I still bear responsibility for subjecting my body to that stress. Perhaps a different mindset would have mitigated the damage. Ultimately, cancer is a confounding malady and the plain truth is that I will never know what caused it. I did absorb the irony that :

> • Had I not had breast cancer they never would have found the lung cancer that surely would have killed me within three years.
> • Had I not had lung cancer they would have started chemo with an unknown severe staph infection already surging through my body.
> • But for lung cancer, my immune system would have been lowered perhaps to a critical level that would have made fighting the staph infection impossible.

My daughter conceived our grandson after my mastectomy and delivered him when the chemo left my system so that it was safe to hold and nuzzle him. My husband and I became closer than we had been in years, and old family splits healed with love and forgiveness. I have been the recipient of abundance and grace. I was gifted with transcendent spiritual experiences that gave me a taste of unitive consciousness. Communities prayed for me. How could I possibly feel anything but fulfilled and fortunate?

Spirit

Medical practitioners and patients are free to reject dealing with issues of the soul. The soul relates to prayer and pleas to a higher power in which some do not believe. When I was diagnosed, I wanted to assess what spiritual claims had the capacity to bring greater health to all levels of my being. When I considered an integral approach to various healing modalities, I was directed to something beyond mind-body medicine. Jeff Levin places this "something" in the categories of "religiousness, spirituality, faith, consciousness, subtle energy, the bioenergy field, non-local mind, our relationship with God" (as cited in Schlitz, p. 283). Larry Dossey's magazine, *Explore: The Journal of Science and Health*, reports on empirical research about the increasing validity of these fascinating avenues to healing.

I needed to replace the "war on cancer" and body-as-machine metaphors with a cyclical, continual, and evolving spiritual focus on my healing. For this I would need an action plan, one that would take courage to enact. It would require that I change certain habits and worldviews, and reassess those of my family's legacy. I was also aware that my medical team might not appreciate my incorporation of spiritual beliefs. How might they react when I reported my spiritual health along with my physical symptoms? Whether they reacted positively or politely ignored me, I was committed to adding spiritual health to my individualized integral healing practice.

Dr. Andrew Weil points out that the symbols for health and healing across cultures always intertwine two opposites. The yin-yang symbol of Taoism and the caduceus (symbolized by the wand of Hermes with intertwined serpents) of Western medicine express perfection when we integrate opposites, and in my case it was that of complementary, alternative, and conventional medical treatments. Regarding the wand of Hermes, Weil explains, power flows freely when complementary opposites are woven into a pattern.

Levin brings spirit directly into the conversation with medicine. He lists a series of phrases that show professionals are reaching beyond the mind-body paradigm to add a spiritual dimension. Whether it is called religiousness, spirituality, faith, consciousness, subtle energy, the bioenergetic field, non-local mind,

216

our relationship with God, or the divine, each of these phrases points to something "beyond" that must be encompassed to describe what it means to be human (as cited in Schlitz, pp. 282-283).

The traditional medical model wanted to treat me as a discrete body, which was a mechanized and reductionist view of who and what I was. The model isolated my disease to a series of body parts, with my care reduced to the separate parts that needed fixing. Biomarkers would serve as the hallmark of my "health." My care would fit into an economics-driven model that relied on high-tech invasive treatment modalities. I was fortunate that Sloan-Kettering never treated me in quite this depersonalized manner. Yet it remained for me to add the spiritual element that would create the synthesis of models I craved. Levin (p. 284) reports that a well-publicized volume of empirical evidence, published under the rubric of "epidemiology of religion," associates religion and spirituality with enhanced health status, physical functioning, and recovery from illness. Magazines such as *Spirituality & Health* and *Explore*, and societies such as the American Institute of Holistic Theology, offer unique perspectives on holistic health and spiritual care.

Healing and the Self (Upper Left)

Thoughts, emotions, and beliefs are now understood to play major roles in healing and illness processes. Studies have found an 18% reduction in mortality for healthy people who attend religious services—better than the 16% rate for colorectal screening. But the same percentage effect as eating more fruits, vegetables, and having a mammography. The placebo effect fits in here, as do meditation, guided imagery, and affirmations.

Healing and the Body (Upper Right)

From the philosophy of science, I came across the term physicalism, which is the view that all factual knowledge can be formulated as a statement about material objects and activities. The language of science reduces people and their illnesses to third-person descriptions of an "It." Doctors must come to see that they

217

are treating more than a biomachine; at the same time, I could not trust anyone who deals with my healing to be ignorant of the very real, very true scientific facts about human anatomy and physiology.

Healing and Culture (Lower Left)

Having a healthcare provider offer positive emotional support can have considerable positive effects on healing. Conversely, there is tyranny of a culture demanding we hold a positive attitude, regardless of our pain level or proignosis. There is no proof that having a positive attitude alone stems tumor growth or that a negative attitude alone encourages tumor growth.

Healing and Systems (Lower Right)

When doctors do not deal with their patients' emotions, people tend to flock to alternative methods—$2 billion is spent annually on a spectrum of complementary and alternative treatments, some specious, some valid. The good news is that two-thirds of American medical schools now incorporate complementary medicine in their curricula. On my web site I have a list of the American medical schools that incorporate holistic systems of healing.

I already had a spiritual practice of meditation, yet when I became ill, I found that it no longer served me—I needed something different that was more specifically directed to my health challenges. Over the years, I created a personalized integral spiritual practice that fits into the Integral Life Practice (ILP) model as described by Wilber and colleagues. The practice covers what I have recounted in this chapter and mirrors ILP's prime modules of Mind, Body, Shadow, Spirit, and Ethics.

My Shadow and Spirit modules were broadened by my two guides to include reading the Tibetan Book of the Dead aloud, both for preparation for a possible imminent death and for the transient deaths we suffer each day. I continue to use Patricia's book on cell-level meditation, and read from the genius of all the world's wisdom traditions. If the practice speaks to me at a particular time, I will use it for my healing. Times of brokenness can be times of wondrous opportunities for growth and innovation that lead to spontaneous
218

spiritual openings. It was now time for me to empty myself of adaptation and to begin to accrue appreciation for where I had been and whatever the future had in store.

PART 3

APPRECIATION

PART 3

APPRECIATION

CHAPTER TWELVE

Entering Contentment

Throughout my rollercoaster ride of lightning strikes, coming to terms with each twist and turn, and adapting to "new normal" conditions, I experienced repeating plateaus of letting go of the "old me." These were times when I released the person who had two cancers, who had no left breast and no left lung lobe, and I could just rest in the simple joy of being alive. I was about to enter a part of the healing cycle called appreciation, which I consider to mean:

Recognition of the quality, value, significance, or magnitude of people and things.
A judgment or opinion, especially a favorable one.
An expression of gratitude.
Awareness or delicate perception, especially of aesthetic qualities or values.
A rise in value or price, especially over time.

But before I could reach an expression of gratitude for the transcendent quality of hope, I had to pass through a plateau of contentment. Achieving satisfaction or present, quiet enjoyment was complicated by my daily physical, psychological, and spiritual challenges.

Physical Challenges

Having a full mastectomy of my left breast meant coming to grips with choosing which prosthetic breast to wear each day. One was the light silicone-bead filled one that rested gently on my sore chest, but did not fill out my clothes as fully as my right breast. The other was the heavy silicone prosthesis that more faithfully twinned my remaining breast, but hurt my shoulder to wear.

Choosing not to have reconstructive surgery meant I no longer could wear lower necklines. My bathing suit with the pocket for me to insert my choice of prosthesis did not look at all attractive, and I have yet to wear it. These physical challenges, as vain as they may sound, prevented me from experiencing contentment.

The thoracotomy presented a more significant physical challenge as it led to almost two years of taking heavy doses of opiates to ameliorate the pain of three surgeries in the same site. The gnawing aches mingled with stabbing jolts of pain were not fertile ground for "quiet satisfaction."

Psychological Challenges

My five months of chemotherapy involved bone pain and extreme digestive discomfort. During this agony I wondered if the treatment agents would search out and destroy every errant cell that had entered my bloodstream through the sentinel node. This critical doubt was enough to crush any sense of quietude or gentle happiness. All I could imagine was more cancer diagnoses over time, more surgeries, and a shortened life.

I eventually stopped reading the blogs sponsored by the various cancer support groups. Roni Caryn Rabin's article, "A Pink-Ribbon Race, Years Long," relates the story of a woman, Dr. Suzanne Herbert, who had metastatic breast cancer. Unfortunately, four percent to six percent of women are at Stage 4 upon their original diagnosis. And 25% of all women who are diagnosed as Stage 1, the smallest, earliest form of cancer, will battle with metastatic disease eventually. The medical establishment does not lay out all of the grim statistics immediately after a woman receives her diagnosis. After my mastectomy, Rick and I sobbed with relief as the gentle Dr. Sacchini told me I was Stage 1, and all I had to do was prevent a recurrence. Only a few weeks later, I was informed I was closer to Stage 2a, since cancer was found in my sentinel node. Therefore my cancer would be more like a chronic illness. "All too often, when people think about breast cancer, they think about it as a problem, it's solved, and you lead a long and normal life; it's a blip on the curve," said Dr. Eric Winer, Director of the Dana-Farber Cancer Institute in Boston, in the above-referenced article. He continued:

> While that's true for many people, each year approximately 40,000 people die of breast cancer—and they all die of metastatic disease. You can see why patients with metastatic disease may feel invisible within the advocacy community.

Those who are at Stage 4 are incurable, even though medical progress permits them to live incrementally longer. The late Elizabeth Edwards survived for several years with metastatic disease; but the median life expectancy is 26 months, and fewer than one in four survive for more than five years. This kind of uncertainty keeps many patients from throwing themselves wholeheartedly into the ethos of hope and empowerment that helps sustain many women with less aggressive forms of the disease.

Dr. Herbert, in the same article, mused that pink ribbon campaigns have raised awareness about breast cancer, but they mask a relentless killer:

> People like the pretty story with the happy ending.... You always hear stories about women who "battled it" and "how courageous" they were. Cancer doesn't care if you're courageous. It's an injustice to all of us who have this. There are women who are no less strong and no less determined to be here, and they'll be dead in two years.

I was shaken after reading the article. How could I create a new framework by which to live my life, and face the physical as well as the psychological challenges that come with cancer?

Spiritual Challenges

I turned to spiritual writers for support and for a renewed sense of appreciation for what I had gained thus far. Alan Cohen, in *Enough Already: The Power of Radical Contentment*, says, "Appreciation is the highest form of prayer, for it acknowledges the presence of good wherever you shine the light of your thankful thoughts." I certainly attempted this form of prayer, as I reached for whatever sense of appreciation I could.

During the time of my three surgeries from November 2010 to January 2011, I attempted as best I could to perform routine "chop wood, carry water" tasks. I also made an effort to take pleasure from every glance at the snow blanketing every surface of my world. Birds flitting to and from our numerous feeders by our back windows thrilled me with their aeronautical swoops, darts, and coordinated flight paths. I surely had mirror neurons that lit up as they flitted within my vision, and I flew along with them in my body-mind.

It took great effort during my treatment period to receive nurturance from touching the earth and letting go of the idea that I am simply a body and with a limited life span. In the words of Buddhist teacher and activist Thich Nhat Hahn:

> I see that this body, made up of the four elements, is not really me and I am not limited by this body. I am part of a stream of life of spiritual and blood ancestors that for thousands of years has been flowing into the present and for thousands of years flows on into the future. I am one with my ancestors. I am one with all people and all beings, whether they are peaceful and fearless or suffering and afraid....The disintegration of this body does not touch me, just as when the plum blossom falls it does not mean the end of the plum tree. I see myself as a wave on the surface of the ocean. My nature is the ocean water. (2003, pp. 168-169)

I accepted this understanding with the humblest and deepest sense of appreciation for the gift of being part of the life process.

Moving Into Appreciation

After the thoracotomy on January 10, 2011, I was engulfed with pain more horrendous than I had ever experienced before. The day after my surgery, with my hospital gown askew, holding onto my IV pole with one hand and my husband's hand in the other, we walked into the hospital's family lounge. There seated across from us was a beautiful woman with red-rimmed eyes. By that time I was familiar with the "privacy dance" of hospital etiquette, where someone wants to unload their grief story but also does not wish to intrude on another's space. After dodging one another's eyes for a while, my husband offered up the cold weather as a conversation opener. It formed a safe platform upon which she could place her grief.

Her 42-year-old daughter lived in Florida with her husband and two young children. Both husband and wife were successful attorneys. After having a lumpectomy and chemotherapy three years prior, she was told there was a large malignant mass wrapped around her sternum. A specialist at Sloan-Kettering was the only one in the country who could safely perform the surgery.

After being sedated, she was awakened, and told that the tumor could not be safely removed. It would remain inside her...growing, giving her three months more to live. Naturally, the mother was in a white-hot state beyond grief.

We spoke and cried together for a long time. Then I went to speak to her daughter for a while. As I became involved in conversation with her (we were both lawyers), my entire body began to move with less agony.

This sad lesson reminded me that there was nothing I could do to tame my errant cells or get them to be orderly or behave in a healthy manner. It was beyond my ability to control them. I had to address new ways of seeing myself that abandoned a search for a "cure." I realized I was no longer covered by any medical protocol where the oncologist could promise "this chemotherapy will reduce your chances of metastases to 10%." I had to be content with the truth that both cancers might metastasize anywhere, at any time, and I would be called into their chaotic dance.

I had been meditating deeply into my body and conversing with my cells.

"Go into a meditative state down into your cells and find that Master Cancer Cell," Patricia prompted during one of our hour-long calls. "Treat it as a second-person 'you' and ask what it needs from you, as odd as that might sound."

Soon I began to get a sense of how it felt and functioned as a voracious and boundary-violating thing, with huge "ego" swelling it to believe that it could take me over and live on through me forever. Like an out of control teen it raged with ugly aggression. I would have to erect a boundary of healthy cells against the infected ones and continue a sort of cell-level dialogue between the cancer-infused and the healthy cells—not to have the healthy ones kill off the cancer cells, but to change their very behavior toward life and away from raging violence. I had to create a different ecology aimed at healing within.

I also saw I would have to make a cultural shift, away from my normal desire to be liked by everyone, and to become more discerning about my memberships. Any group would have to welcome me and understand who I was at my core, and not trigger a stress reaction. This discernment would save me from being drawn into our cultural mandate of ignoring personal needs in favor of adapting to the demands of the group. Unfortunately, this was not a lesson I learned until after treatment ended, so ingrained was the cultural mandate to fit into a particular style of awareness and of my culture's shadow.

Thich Nhat Hahn laid down the foundation for my nascent ability to be appreciative of my condition at this moment, and the moments thereafter: "When conditions are sufficient we manifest and when conditions are not sufficient we go into hiding. It's as simple as that." By hiding, this Buddhist author meant that birth and death are but notions; they are not real. I concentrated for weeks on his premise that once we understand that there is no permanent self, that I would not be destroyed if I died of my cancers, I would be able to approach my numerous challenges with a sense of appreciation. I took his book, *No Death, No Fear*, along with me wherever I went for days, along with Sharon Salzberg's book, *Faith*.

Salzberg, a Buddhist meditation teacher, understood that we are

226

a meaning-making species, and we interpret our own fragmented experiences into narratives that can explain and map them. Unfortunately, some narratives lock us into fragments that we mistakenly interpret as the whole, whereas other narratives reveal the whole, relationships, and connection with the All.

I was perhaps genetically predisposed to be a mystic, but my family locked me into those negative fragments that I was told represented the All. I believed that my problem was me at my core, and thus there was no way out for me. I had very little reason to have faith in myself or believe I could change my life. There was the "Curse of the Greenbergs," which my mother had taught me would be there to sour my own predestined fate. When my mother wrote of the horrors and grief of her family back to her great-grandmother's life down to her own misery, she told me that my chapter of suffering was going to be written next.

I lived out that narrative for 64 years. How did I make that magnificent and major change from believing I was destined to suffer to believing I had the ability to change my life, and to live a life free of suffering? It was through integral spirituality, and a belief in the impermanence of the physical body in the face of the permanence of Spirit.

When the legendary, nihilistic figure of Mara set out to dissuade Siddhartha, soon to evolve into the Buddha, from his attempt to become enlightened, Mara chose to attack Siddhartha's belief in his own potential. Siddhartha resolved this dualistic tension by asking the earth to bear witness to his right to be sitting under the bodhi tree, his right to aspire to full understanding and infinite compassion. With he woke the next morning, he was enlightened.

I have the right to be happy. No genetic disposition, no ancestral curse, can interrupt that right. I can envision a better life for myself, and for you. Thus is faith admitted into our world. Faith is a verb in Pali, Latin, and Hebrew. It is something we must do. It is the willingness to take the next step. And where will that next step take us? Into the darkness, into the unknown. It is a journey, not a destination; faith takes us into an unknown land where we must risk it all. What must we give up in this journey? The firm belief that we are in an unchanging place that will stay as is, for our security. Where am I on this journey with faith? I choose life. I align myself with the potential inherent in my life. I give myself over to that potential.

Phase of Appreciation

The winter after my surgeries was very strange for the Mid-Atlantic region. We'd never had so much snow. The whipping winds snapped towering trees that crashed down onto unsuspecting houses and flattened cars. The chill came and stayed, and we could only dream of the time when we could fling off our salt-crusted Uggs.

Why mention the weather? It is a state experience that we might merge with and feel one with the manifest realm. Wilber writes, "I no longer witness the clouds, I am the clouds; I do not hear the rain, I am the rain; I can no longer touch the earth, for I am the earth...." What a test for me! Do not flinch from the icy blast as I exit the car, for I am one with the icy blast. I will also be the crocus daring to poke its precious bud above the snowline.

But I am also that Witness who will disappear and reflect back on these manifestations as an empty mirror, rather than being any one of them as self/other. , What lesson do I learn from being in this body/mind and using cancer for serious spiritual growth ? I have a body, but I am not that body.

Why then do I manage to care about the affirmations, visualizations, and meditations, plus the chemo, the 10 daily pills, the cautious eating, and Purell hand washing in which I mindfully engaged while in treatment? Patanjali, who lived in the 2nd century B.C. and compiled the Yoga Sutras, wrote that if we identify the Witness solely with the subjects and objects of our daily awareness, we create a state of bondage. Was I in bondage, then? I can, by grace or spiritual practice, achieve identity with the Witness and the awareness that I am bound with all of creation. Once my conscious awareness of being the All has been unveiled, or felt, I don't need to act through my will, since the right action becomes an immediate, natural, and simple step for me to take.

That is all fine and well to study intellectually, but I still struggled with the idea of my own death. There I was, in my mid-sixties, not young but not too old to die, heaven knows. Did I expect special dispensation from fate? What I did feel badly about was that I had, at last and with great effort, rewoven and healed my ego's terrible wounds, and achieved a new sense of self and tranquility. The scars left from my dysfunctional upbringing and trauma-filled life had ceased to attack me when similar events presented themselves. I had forgiven my mother for her actions stemming from her illness, and honored and loved her unconditionally. I was in a loving relationship with Melissa, who I am so proud to call my daughter today as she serves with grace and dignity as a wife, mother, and nurse.

And yet I remain one mammogram or scan away from terror and creeping fear. The cycles of healing would have to begin all over again. Was there some manner of interrupting the terror and fear, and maintaining a state of appreciation longer and turning it into an entire stage of living moment to moment?

As I worked and meditated with Lorraine and Patricia at different, I discovered the identity I had created via nurture was that Lynne Suffers. My life had been framed as one prolonged yet segmented tale of suffering, of unjust victimization and outrageous assaults. What they had me do, so brilliantly, was to rid myself of the cloak I had worn for 64 years.

I visualized greeting that sad self, and as she approached me I had nothing but loving compassion for her, how she struggled against the role she had to inhabit to win the acceptance of her family. I held her close to my heart, and turned away from her as I walked back into my freed Self. I looked over my shoulder to see her sad and beaten countenance smile slightly at my receding back. And I walked back into the radiant Emptiness, exiting the bardo.

The term is from the *Tibetan Book of the Dead*. "Bardo" literally means a period of time between two events, and it should be apparent that this is precisely where I was situated, leaving one bardo for another. What I aimed to take out of the bardo of illness and into appreciation of my new normal included understandings about life, death, impermanence, and not knowing. I am comfortable with silence, always have been, as an only child. But now I can discern when my anxiety creeps up to prod me to "make someone else comfortable" at my own expense and in opposition to my own honest needs.

I no longer feel the need to sacrifice myself for any "other"; I have held the glory of what I am without fiction. I deserve to be alive—yes, that simple admission has been a huge issue for me all my life. I can offer much to others now from the clarity of my natural existence. I am the vehicle through which I offer to we, to you, and all of you. I have had superb guidance from Patricia and Lorraine. I no longer feel the need to sacrifice myself for any "other"; I have held the glory of what I am without fiction or cosmetic application to enhance or obfuscate a perceived detraction. I have had my dear friend with whom I wrestle into freedom from error and mistake, Robin. I have had Rick, my husband of 42 years, and a masterful cheerleader whom I have come to appreciate more than ever. I have an incredibly kind and ethical daughter, Erica, and her loving husband, Simon. I made subtle level contact with my grandson in utero. Adam exited his uterine bardo on July 28, 2011, to join our loving family and is now a boundlessly cheerful toddler; and little puppy soul Chloe, the best companion I could have wished for during the months of my illness and treatment.

Yes, I survived an unbelievable journey with as much fortitude as I could. Yes, I developed coping strategies to reign in an emotional catharsis, and it was high time that such a cathartic outburst was permitted. Yes, my limit had been reached, and I had to respect that fact. I could endure no more. My chemotherapy ended on July 11, 2011, the day before my 66th birthday and on that next day I broke open again. I could not stop crying, wrenching and jerking convulsions of tears flooding down my cheeks. My heart once again had softened with appreciation and gratitude for my body-mind for enduring what it had tolerated. Social worker Frances E. Englander says that during times of brokenness we are reliving aspects of our histories that have been painful, traumatic, and overwhelming (as cited in Taylor, 2008, p. 7). That fit me perfectly, and permitted my appreciation of what my soul felt compelled to expel in the form of pain and tears.

Lightning Strike Four

I smiled my way through November 2011's scan without even needing Rick to keep me company. Two days later I saw Dr. Graham, and inquired as to the health and rambunctiousness of her two boys. I then sat still as I awaited her assurance that I was fine once again. I did not receive it, nor did I get any pleasantries about what the scan showed. When I took my seat, she was not smiling.

"Lynne, there is a supraclavical lymph node on your left side that the radiologist has been monitoring for three months. Apparently it has grown substantially since July and you will need a biopsy."

"What is it, for God's sake? Haven't I been tormented enough?" My tranquility, equanimity, and quiet gratitude quickly dissipated.

She reached over to grab my hands. "We won't know, but there are three possibilities. First, it could be metastatic breast cancer. If so, we will treat it as aggressively as possible. Or it could be metastatic lung cancer."

"What's the third possibility?" I asked in a familiar foggy brew of disbelief and horror.

"It could be nothing," she offered without conviction. She scooted her chair closer to me so that our knees touched. "Look, Lynne, if it is a metastasis from the breast cancer, we will do more surgery, radiation, and more chemo. But it puts your life expectancy at about five years."

"And if it is from the lung cancer?" I asked, knowing this would be the worst-case scenario.

"If it is from the lung, Lynne, there are always clinical trials and I'll make sure you get into all you qualify for." In other words, I would be terminal.

If ever I felt that cell-level meditation had value and worth, this was the time to dig in with more conscious intentionality than I had ever attempted previously. I worked the meditation over and over, deeper and deeper, and put more faith (there's that word again) into the process. I usually started meditation just hoping, but not entirely convinced, that it would have some effect. I'm a political scientist/rationalist/lawyer who came to spiritual and transformative work only in my forties, rather than in my teens or twenties, as so many others who have written about their own paths. I never stayed at an ashram or had a guru; I never went to a long meditation retreat or bolted off to India. I always felt as though I was playing catch-up spiritually.

On Thursday of the lymph node biopsy week, once again prior to Thanksgiving, my husband and I were once again at Sloan-Kettering. I dressed in a gown, had an IV put into the port that had been implanted into my right chest wall, and was wheeled into the operating room. The surgeon went through her little speech:

"I'm going to make three incisions to get as much of the lymph node as possible, since we don't know if this is lung or breast cancer..."

"Or it's nothing, right?"

"Uh, sure," she stated dismissively.

She began going back and forth over the area where the lymph node was located with an ultrasound wand, but I couldn't see because my left side was draped. I felt the wand stop and then proceed up my neck. Then she paused. She spoke softly to her assistant and asked for the surgeon who had just finished up in the operating suite next to mine.

He entered, and they shared a whispered conversation as I began to drift off. He then held the wand and I felt him going back and forth over my clavicle. He paused, and then I felt him go up my neck. Then there was total silence.

He lifted the drape from my face and said, "I suggest that you go home and buy a lottery ticket. Today is your lucky day. The lymph node has disappeared entirely."

I was wheeled back into my room where my husband looked at me with alarm. I had not been gone that long for the biopsy to be executed. I really did not know how to articulate what had just happened, so I drew his head to my mouth and whispered, "There is no lymph node. It's gone."

Rick and I could not bring ourselves to speak as I dressed. We both left in a daze, and yes, we did buy a lottery ticket, and no, I did not win money. The next day I had to get a prescription from Sloan-Kettering. Dr. G heard I was there, and flew out of her office and hugged me tightly twice with tears in her eyes. When I asked if she'd like to analyze the results, she shook her head vigorously, "No!"

That is why I have faith, and dare I say it, more trust. I have gone through a sea change, it is true. But I will never know if or whether the disease will reassert its miserable, self-destructive presence. The Integral framework has provided me with a way to hold the enormity of what I have experienced, and faith that I can hold whatever comes along in the future. None of us get out of this journey alive—I am aware of that deeply and openly.

The central part of appreciation is a leap past hope. As a child I memorized and clung to Emily Dickinson's phrases:

> Hope is the thing with feathers
> That perches in the soul
> And sings the tune without the words
> And never stops at all

I have come to understand her poem from a different perspective today. Yes, the soul sings "hope" without cease, since that is something we believe will carry us over the most turbulent waters. Even when the doctor thought I had a metastatic lymph node, she spoke of the hope that I might live longer than five years or that a new treatment would emerge. I found "hope" to be a dry and lifeless presence in my mouth at that time. It sounded childlike to me. Then I came across a quote by Margaret Mitchell, author of *Gone With The Wind*, who wrote, "Life's under no obligation to give us what we expect. We take what we get and are thankful it's no worse than it is." And this idea seemed to fit my reality with ultimate truth. I needed to find something that permitted me to go beyond hope.

CHAPTER THIRTEEN

Transcending Hope

In the quieter times between my lightning strikes, I had the presence to be humble and appreciative of the opportunities for grace I had been given. My diagnosis occurred near Erica's birthday. Working backward we determined she became pregnant on the date of my mastectomy. Little Adam was born exactly two weeks after my chemo ended so I could cuddle him. I find it difficult even now to spell out what all of this might mean, or if it is just a series of random inkblots I've tried to assemble into a pattern.

I have, nonetheless, undergone, tolerated, endured, and held up under extraordinary challenges. I have received blessings and awakenings to Spirit I never would have assumed possible. I also purposefully entered a time of respite from the fall of 2012 through the fall of 2013. Respite comes from the Latin word for "respect." I needed to repair myself and to postpone any vestige of frenetic activity in order to respect the sacred changes going on within my body. This does not make me special or distinctive. It was just not part of my upbringing to respect my internal needs, and thus I engaged in a long overdue period of self-nurturance.

It is crushing for me to admit that but for the two cancers, I might not have awakened to this holy need, and would have continued on a course of frenetic activity toward some ego-framed ending. Among the many reasons for this respite, this retreat of body, mind, and spirit, was to metabolize and reconnect with an extraordinary experience I had when fighting the cellulitis infection and fearing the lung cancer would kill me. But it is a difficult experience to discuss. It also poses difficulties in attempting to crystallize in language an ineffable experience. It is far easier to describe the medical findings that led to yet another "incidental" life-saving call than to describe how it was received in my gut, and what emotions fairly exploded along with the medical finding.

I am in a space I have never been before, a place of luminosity, gratitude, quietude, and rest. My engine is no longer revving up at exaggerated RPMs to prove that I deserve to be alive. I breathe, therefore I am. It bears repeating: I do not have the need or ability to scuttle crab-like hither and yon, nor to extend myself beyond my smaller self. Cancer bore me to this place, as odd as that might seem. My birth in July and thus my "horoscope destiny" of being represented by Cancer the Crab somehow delivered me to a soft, restful nest where I need to be, quietly, as I expand, healthy cells to healthy cells, into new spaces that will offer my Self as best I can, in peace, authenticity, and love, by just breathing in and out.

There is a certain degree of courage in looking into a mirror and seeing one's own face, says Dzogchen Ponlop, a leading Tibetan Buddhist scholar and writer. But our journey starts at that very reflection, and I am reminded that this raw reflection must not be compromised by drawing cosmetic changes onto a mirror, for once we move our head a centimeter, the changes stay behind on the mirror, but not on our real selves.

It has been traumatic and testing for me to do just that—to look at my reflection with compassion instead of negative judgment. Others may see an idealized reflection in their own imaginations, and decide that an ugly reflection must be an error on someone else's part. But there is no external source to create that raw reflection, and getting a cleaner mirror or better lighting will not solve the problem. It is the curse and the gift that we see ourselves as we truly are in that mirror. It is at our own command that we begin the journey of working with this reflection of our minds and our actions. And thus it began for me in November 2010 while in a walking meditative state, IV pole in hand, around the corridor of my floor at Sloan-Kettering.

It came during a period of self-pity as I catalogued what my death within 18 months would deprive me of enjoying. I would miss my adult students. I would miss knowing my grandchild. I would miss the first crocus of spring and the overwhelming fragrance of the hyacinths. I would miss my home and husband, daughter and close circle of friends. But this bout of self-pity smacked too much of ego, and I realized I had to turn my attention to my higher self.

I went into a deep meditative state as I trudged with IV pole in my right hand, and then "looked" around me. I "saw" my "self" walk up to two huge mahogany doors. I tried as hard as I could to push them open, since I "knew" somehow that beyond those doors was death, and it was my time to surrender and enter that domain. Try as I might, I could not push the doors open. I saw my "self" as a small creature attempting this herculean task. And then—as I walked around and around the corridors, I let each prize go…just go…until I had fallen so deeply that all was spaceless space and timeless time.

Suddenly I was no longer that small Lynne-self. Instead, I had grown to an unfathomable dimension and floated off into the void that now surrounded me. To paraphrase one excellent description of this sensation, my thoughts and self-pity moved by grace so far into the background of my self-sense as I continued to stand upright and move around the corridors, until they totally disappeared. Without being able to identify my "self" with my thought-stream, all attachment to self-pity or any other emotion vanished as well. My body continued to weave through the oncoming stream of patients, visitors, and nurses, but the movement was done without thought or conscious control.

At that moment my field of vision appeared to encompass all of creation. I became aware of a limitless dimension that I had experienced by grace several times in the past, but was unable to hold onto for more than a few weeks. I was resting in, and as, boundless empty space:

In that empty space, the mind is completely still; there is no time, no memory, not even a trace of personal history. And the deeper you fall into that space, the more everything will continue to fall away, until finally all that will be left is you. When you let absolutely everything go—body, mind, memory and time—you will find, miraculously, that you still exist. In fact, in the end, you discover that all that exists is you! (Cohen, 2012, p. 9).

I inhabited an unmanifest domain that was "unchanging, beginningless, and endless". It is what I have come to know as the Ground of Being, or the Divine; I might call it God as well. And then I began to laugh, a hearty, loving, full-throated laugh of cosmic humor for the "am-ness" that I occupied. And within this no-place that is the beginning of all places we might occupy, I turned back toward my very real hospital room.

Joy-filled, I looked toward the space above my door. There I found a golden infinity sign glowing above the loving yet strong-willed faces of my father and my mother. Their visages communicated that they would not let anything harm me. I was protected and deeply loved. I understood what needed to be comprehended and there was no rush to do or to be. I phoned Patricia and told her that there was nothing more to say; I was healed in the only sense that I needed to be healed.

This state experience lasted for months but was finally disrupted by the excruciating pain that I experienced after the thoracotomy. I do not rue the end of that state; rather, it is something I know is more real than the experience I am having this instant as I type these words. I know that I can access that reality when I go so deep that there is but One, and I Am That.

Integral Optimism

I was back at *adaptation* as I tried to integrate this numinous experience into my understanding of all the phases of healing. Then I finally realized what Patricia meant when she instructed me to get to know my Master Cancer Cell. When I slipped back into a less complete healing phase, I wondered what I could carry with me for support? What truth did I possess that would educate me for the journeys and phases to come?

And then it came to me: Cancer thinks it is God. It colonizes itself from one primordial Master Cancer Cell to billions... and then it evolves! As chemotherapy destroys the breast cancer cells, some that are more adapted to survival and growth can mutate, evade the toxins, and nest in organs, tissues, or bones far from their primal beginnings. That is the ever-present fear. They learn our tricks to destroy them and then find ways to continue to procreate.

I finally understood what my Master Cancer Cell was demanding. Cancer is the pathology of excess, the expansionist disease, setting up colonies and raping the natives. Mukherjee (2010) states, "It lives desperately, inventively, fiercely, territorially, cannily, and defensively—at times, as if teaching us how to survive. To confront cancer is to encounter a parallel species, one perhaps more adapted to survival than even we are." I thought of science fiction movies, with enemies depicted as crab-like segmented figures arcing up to fire at the small and vulnerable humans. I thought of "Alien" and its progeny.

Mukherjee helps us understand our current cultural landscape in dealing with cancer as he adds a history and linguistic analysis of the terms as they morphed over time. The dreaded word cancer comes from Hippocrates around 400 B.C., when we see his first mention in medical literature of "karkinos," the Greek word for "crab," denoting cancer as a name for the disease. The tumor he observed had a body of swollen blood vessels around it, which reminded Hippocrates of a crab dug in the sand with its legs spread in a circle. Some cancer sufferers of that era felt as though a crab were moving under their flesh as the disease spread stealthily. This burden being carried about the body brought along a second linguistic association: onkos, Greek for load or burden, both physical and psychological, from which we derived "oncology."

Skipping ahead to medicine around the World Wars and then into the Cold War, the cancer researchers of modernity hit on a military theme for a Manhattan Project prototype that would "kill" the steadily increasing diagnoses of this horrific disease. We were at war. We needed an all-out attack plan. And in the forefront of our troops we had the heroes, the doctors! They were the Eisenhowers, MacArthurs, Pattons and Deweys of the war on cancer. There was one enemy, there was one cancer, and the heroes could certainly track it to its roots and vanquish it with a nuclear weapon.

238

But such was not to be the case. Cancer appeared as hundreds of variants around a common theme. Cancers possessed temperaments, personalities—even individualized behaviors. Yet the medical establishment stuck to the belief that there was a one-size-fits-all treatment. One approach to attacking cancer was expected to fit all of the different carcinomas; this was the predominant worldview within the medical establishment even as patients came in with cancers of the appendix, tongue, and tonsil, in addition to invasions of every conceivable bone, tissue, or organ.

With the advent of chemotherapy in the 1980s, it became obvious that combinations of toxic drugs had to be infused, since a one-strike, deep surgical attack did nothing much to extend life. Linking these extensive and mutilating surgical attacks with infusions of toxic chemicals took on what Mukherjee refers to as "total hell."

Yet little by little, cancer by cancer, drug combination by drug combination, we began to see cancer patients in the 1960s showing signs that they could remain cancer-free. The doyenne of cancer philanthropy, Mary Lasker, made liberal use of the moon landing in 1969 as the propulsive thrust to her "War On Cancer," which hit the national media December 9, 1969. She used her wealth and media savvy to agitate President Nixon to create a NASA-like organization that could supervise the battle against cancer.

Gone were the days of whispering about the "Big C"; from Solzhenitsyn's *Cancer Ward* to "Brian's Song" to "Love Story," cancer had insinuated itself into popular culture as stealthily as it did into healthy cells. The enemy was within us, marauding, unheralded until such time as the system could no longer take the assault. The scalpel and the radical mastectomy were the heralded weapons wielded by the heroes of the war, hacking away at the cruel enemy within.

By 1981, however, the entire metaphor of combat had fallen into disrepute. To some, the heroes were butchering women; chemotherapy trials were destructive and sadistic. The doctors fell back into being scientists looking at the data, if they dared—for the data did not prove their hypotheses. We now recognize that the story of cancer is not really the story of doctors who struggle to survive:

It is the story of patients who struggle and survive, moving from one embankment of illness to another. Resilience, inventiveness, and survivorship—qualities often ascribed to great physicians—are reflected qualities, emanating first from those who struggle with illness and only then mirrored by those who treat them. (Mukharjee, 2010, p. 111)

To those who came before me such as Treya Kilam Wilber, to those who endured 10 to 12 vomiting sessions every day during their treatment, to those who went under the scalpel numerous times in an attempt to root out evil, I bow down to them for their suffering. It is because of them that I can sit at my computer and do what I wish to do today. I am so deeply grateful for their sacrifices, courage, and commitment to life when none could promise it to them.

I do not know how long I will continue to live "cancer free," but I am fortunate to have had the experience of entering a blissful state for a while, even if I could not maintain it. I found that within this "time without time" and "space without space," everything is possible. I had only joy surrounding me and nothing could ultimately happen to me. After resting in appreciation for several months, the intense pain of the lung cancer surgery caused me to slip back into coming to terms and then phase into adaptation. All I could do was to lean into the pain, and through it. My test would be whether I could continue to rest in appreciation after all I had been through thus far. Looking back over my life from my earliest memories, all I can touch is pain, frustration, and lack of security. Here with my health crises I encountered these three fearsome companions again, making my life an endless stream of anguish. Where was my safety to be when I could slide out of a blissful state back to a partial and non-integrated one? The poet Rumi beautifully answers this query:

Your Worth

You know the value of every article of merchandise,
But if you don't know the value of your own soul,
It's all foolishness.
You've come to know the fortunate and the
inauspicious stars,
But you don't know whether you yourself
Are fortunate or unlucky.

This, this is the essence of all sciences—
That you should know who you will be
When the Day of Reckoning arrives.

This poses the question, but does not answer who I will be when my day of reckoning arrives. Am I bounded by the "Curse of the Greenbergs?" Haunted by the people who scapegoated me and left me bereft of self-confidence? Surrounded by events that cast me into unrelenting despair over decades? Or was there a way for me to look at my life's trajectory and remain optimistic within a realistic context?

I took the term "integral optimism" from a speech on global issues and applied it to the context of those with serious diagnoses:

In the face of my dire personal challenge, I am obliged to cultivate my highest spiritual awareness. How can I go through the cancer dance unless I am aware that fundamentally I am One, as Self, as All-Pervading Spirit? If I am not aware of this truth, then I will not be able to concentrate on right action or right thought, and thus I will suffer psychologically and spiritually.

I am obliged to build a bridge between my sense of being a separate, concrete self and the knowledge that I am also founded upon and within an absolute Self. This is an integral "both/and" approach that supported me throughout my journey with its harsh physical and psychological pain.

If I wish to avoid the term "cancer victim," there is an alternative one being used in some areas: "cancer thriver." Although it might seem to be a precious term, it has a purpose of directing my attention to the now and tomorrow's now. I have a finite time upon this earth in my precious human life, and I am obliged to make the most of my potential and my passions for the good of the All.

I am obliged not to fall into the duality of naïve optimism or depressing despair. I have shown various shifts between these two polarities over the months while my major thrust has been to keep a more balanced sense of what my illness might mean for my future. "Not-knowing" was the only sane way of looking into my crystal ball, but I had flashes at both extremes.

Integral optimism has to be something I could breathe into, every moment of every day from here on out. The irony is that the freedom I received came from contemplating my own death—not by repressing or avoiding the possibility on our fundamental mortality.

Burt Parlee, the author, then quoted Tibetan Lama Anagarika Govinda:

> If one doesn't meditate on death in the morning, one's morning is wasted. If one doesn't meditate on death in the afternoon, one's afternoon is wasted. If one doesn't meditate on death in the evening, one's evening is wasted. In just this way, most people waste their entire lives. (Parlee, 2010)

Baby Boomers might find it difficult to do what the Lama suggests. I found it difficult to absorb this wisdom at first as well. My friends were going for facelifts, tummy tucks, Botox injections, and exotic facials—all manner of youth-sustaining measures. I have no quarrel with efforts to fend off Father Time, yet eventually these measures cannot mask the natural processes underneath, and contemplating death must enter the picture. None of us gets out of here alive, regardless of our religious beliefs.

Then where is the hope? I could not promise myself life after 18 months when the radiologist thought I had small cell lung cancer; Dr. G could not promise me more than five years' more life when she thought I had metastatic lung cancer; and I cannot promise my family that I'll be present at our next gathering. We know that life is finite; we just do not know when our time will end in this manifestation. That sounds hopeless.

But once we admit to ourselves that we are of Spirit / God / Goddess / the Divine, then we are touching our true identities. Once that realization is integrated into our body/minds, we know where we can put our trust and that trust will never be violated. Something beyond mere hope begins to take form. If an individual with cancer cannot come to that ultimate realization, the sense of optimism will evaporate with the next worrisome blood test or scan.

The Spectrum of Optimism

What happens when our desire to be hopeful collides with the indignity of a cancer diagnosis? Our very sense of identity is challenged along with our sense of what we believe, our worldview, and our perception of the future. Integral healing envelops continuums, developmental and evolutionary models, and the spectrum of optimism fits in perfectly. I found the following to be a fairly typical representation of the continuum of integral optimism, first introduced by Parlee in the context of global issues:

Apocalyptic Pessimism: Some who have been diagnosed with cancer tilt toward an "end of the world" scenario. They interpret their cancer as caused by the rape of Gaia, despoliation of the planet, or chemical additives to the entire food supply and all of us are therefore vulnerable to similar fates.

Paranoid Pessimism: Some cancer victims believe that "Big Pharma" and agricultural conglomerates have poisoned the earth and are responsible for cancer. Big Pharma purposely keeps known cures away from sufferers in order to retain profits—this belief is prevalent in a surprising number of books, blogs, and Internet sites.

Worried Pessimism: Looking at life from a victim mentality, these people cannot conceive of things looking up for them or other cancer sufferers. They recount stories of all the people they have heard about who succumbed to the illness. This reminded me of my mother's constant fear of contracting cancer, or of conflating a minor skin cancer with fulminating carcinomas.

Cautious Optimist: These cancer patients have a more balanced view of their diagnosis. Although they know that the battle ahead will be a great challenge, there is the hope that they will survive, and they read books and share stories with others who have beaten the disease and have gone on for decades to live out their lives.

Inspired Optimist: The person diagnosed with cancer at this level of the continuum challenges established maxims associated with the disease and reaches beyond what seems possible. One such woman scheduled her radical mastectomy around her normal activities and believed that her surgery would be as troublesome as having a root canal, perhaps even less painful.

Idealistic Optimist: The Idealists believe that by choosing the right hospital/surgeon/procedure/holistic entity, they will definitely recover and have no further issues. Although I had great support from the Integral model, I never presumed that it was a magic bullet that guaranteed survival.

Naive Optimism: I know those who, after feeling a lump in their breast or experiencing difficulty breathing or bleeding from an orifice, refuse to seek medical intervention for a diagnosis for fear of what might be revealed. Some have already been diagnosed and refuse to abide by any sensible protocol, choosing instead to believe the magical "Cancer Healing Secrets Your Doctor Doesn't Want You to Know," which is often followed by an ad to buy a magic elixir. Then there is the belief in thinking happy thoughts and trusting in the Lord (or belief system of your choice). No study has indicated that any of these pre-rational beliefs is effective.

Integral optimism: In contrast, this level involves striving surrender, which is where I chose to embed my dance with cancer. Parlee explains his interaction of seeming opposites as follows:

> Combining the opposites of striving and surrender, we arrive at a place that is at once sober, spiritually grounded, positively engaged, "unreasonably" ambitious, and yet realistic and open to whatever may come. (Parlee, 2010)

When I was faced with the possibility of a painful death within 18 months, I realized I had to spend every minute striving to survive, but to gracefully surrender to my mortality if that is what emerged as my destiny.

Cancer seemed to follow me from birth. Being a July baby, I fell under the "sign" of Cancer—a shameful thing to admit during the Age of Aquarius. During the 1970s and 1980s, I would rework my discomfort in having to reveal my birth sign. I couldn't claim to be a more presentable Aries the Ram, Taurus the Bull, Gemini the Twins, Leo the Lion, and so on: I was a feared disease or a nasty pincer in a hardened carapace. In all fairness, though, let me note that Scorpio is a Scorpion, and Libra is the only inanimate sign of the zodiac. But still, cancer?

"I am a Moon Child," I would coyly respond. Far better to be perceived as a "luna-tic" than a carcinoma. But since I have had cancer within me, I have begun to look at the sign of Cancer in another sense: I began to consider that I was not only born under the sign of Cancer, but that I had been bourne under the sign of cancer as well. From The Collaborative International Dictionary of English, two definitions of "bourne" resonated with me:

1. To possess mentally; to carry or hold in the mind; to entertain; to harbor; and
2. To endure; to tolerate; to undergo; to suffer.

I am certainly not happy that I had to undergo this series of bodily, emotional and spiritual assaults. Had I a hand in the decision, I certainly would have turned the "opportunity" away. But I have at last been able to understand the puzzling and dazzling patterns of my life as I have been borne by the encounter with cancer, which permitted me to make my life a sacred journey.

Cancer was no "gift" for me, as some writers have relayed, yet I had been carried along to discover worlds within myself previously untapped and unknown. I believe it is this sense of the disease that provokes so many authors to describe the transcendent impact cancer has had on them. In law, we use the legal term "but for" (e.g., but for the negligence of the parents, the child would not have been injured; but for the man driving drunk, there would not have been a catastrophic collision). In my case, but for the cancer, I would not have adopted the striving surrender approach to life.

Mukherjee applies the metaphors up to our current age:

> We tend to think of cancer as a "modern" illness because its metaphors are so modern. It is a disease of overproduction, of fulminant growth—growth unstoppable, growth tipped into the abyss of no control.... Cancer is that machine unable to quench its initial command (to grow) and thus transformed into an indestructible, self-propelled automaton. (Mukherjee, 2010)

He quotes Susan Sontag in *Illness as Metaphor* when she cites tuberculosis as the illness of the 19th century. Cancer, he argues, is our metaphor in this age of desperate individualism. The origin of the dreaded word metastasis is a curious mix—"beyond stillness" in Latin—an unmoored, partially unstable state that captures the peculiar instability of modernity. My busy-ness, my need to produce in order to feel that I have a valid place on earth, is certainly congruent with this concept. To be still, to meditate, take long walks in nature, just quietly play with my grandson—is that a waste of time, or is it the opposite of metastasis, a sign of health and stability? That was my challenge in surrendering into stillness.

Transcendent Hope

Going beyond hope when one faces a critical illness might first seem sorrowful. Who would want to go beyond hope in times of stress and serious doubt when to embrace hope can be a wish-fulfilling, magical thinking panacea by which to escape dire predictions? I had this difficult task given my family's propensity to embrace the negative at every opportunity. When my mother came to visit with me and sat in the kitchen, her food requests would be delivered thusly: "You wouldn't have [name the food stuff], would you." Not a question. A statement. Conditional, yes, yet with a negative inflection so acidic that I took to simply declaring "no" in retaliation.

It took me years of reconditioning to be open to hope, which I believed to be a totally irrational response to the vicissitudes of my life. Add to that our cultural propensity to surround every statement with a statistic. In some of the articles I read, I have a 25% chance of dying from a metastasis of one of my two cancers. How does hope fit in with the quantification of every aspect of our lives? When Dr. G thought I had a metastatic lymph node, she told me there was always hope that a new treatment or drug might come along. Hope can sound irrational, and is often relegated to that "unscientific" part of our lives: religion and spirituality.

The subject of hope is located in the near or far future: winning an athletic contest or getting good news from a CAT scan. And it is uniformly positive if it pertains to the self or a loved one. Peter

Heszler classifies hope as irrational, immanent, or transcendent. Immanent hope derives from our individual quest to win, run faster, sell more products to make more money; it comes from the materialistic sphere of our lives where hope is usually considered beneficial (Heszler).

Conversely, "transcendent hope" comes from the religious or spiritual spheres of life. Regardless of the variations among the wisdom traditions, Heszler notes one very deep and important feature that they all share:

> There is a hope for the divine and the human to be unified: when the "karma" is diminished (Hinduism), when one gets to "nirvana" (Buddhism), when the Messiah comes (Judaism), when Christ rules at the end of times (Christianity), etc. For religious people this hope (faith) is a basic, orientation point of life. Let us call this hope transcendent hope, since the subject of hope (the divine part) lies outside of this world. (Ibid)

The difference between immanent hope and transcendent hope, he notes, is the length of the arrows, but the source is the same.

Transcendent hope is not necessarily tied to a particular outcome, and is not tied to any effort by humans to get the "correct" desired result. Rather, it is hope grounded in an overwhelming sense of presence of the divine, however one conceives of it. There is a sense of a profoundly larger force at work in, through, and around the humans involved.

This is not fragile optimism, the smiley-faced icon of merchandising, or the perfunctory "Have a nice day." Fragile optimism is accompanied by a sense of entitlement, and thus when the desired result does not happen, there can be a sense of profound guilt or rejection.

The relevance of a transcendent hope may sometimes be that of the "spring in the desert". If, in a desert region, water can be found it is because in some distant and unknown place incalculable quantities of water have sunk into the ground and disappeared. Only because of that infiltration in some distant place, continuing over a long time and developing pressure in a stratum of porous rock, can water be carried under the desert soil. Far away, it is can be found as a seemingly miraculous source of sustenance. (Yoder, 1971)

For me, transcendent hope is best articulated as integral optimism, and it comes from the Source of all Being. I cannot merely rest in bliss assuming the cancer will evaporate. I must take affirmative steps toward working with Spirit and natural processes to manifest the healing process. For this, I created Integral Healing Practice.

CHAPTER FOURTEEN

Integral Healing Practice

With no sense of irony or comedy intended, perhaps the best way to approach a diagnosis of cancer is to call oneself a "cancer dancer."

When this phrase popped into my consciousness, I recoiled to think of cancer with its tentacled, deformed arms around me in a formal dancing embrace. But when I stopped to inquire why that phrase resonated the more I sat with it, I came to see the phrase as pointing to being in a relationship. I was certainly in a relationship with my cancer cells after diagnosis and during treatment. The cells might well now be destroyed by the chemotherapy, yet I was aware that at any time a sleeper cell might decide to awake and "turn" other healthy cells against what is "me."

But in a much larger sense, if a cell begins to mutate, it still is me, and the next step is to embrace all of my cells, including the cancer cells, as Patricia had me do. I asked what the cancer cells wanted from me and what I could learn from them. There is a practice known as Big Mind, an offshoot of the psychological practice of voice dialog that has been infused with Zen and integral perspectives. The process begins with a trained facilitator who asks to speak to our "Controller," which is the prime director that protects our "selves" in their numerous guises. The facilitator asks this voice's permission to speak to the other voices within, such as the voice of the Wounded Child or the Victim. In a sense, this is what I learned to do with Patricia: "Will the Facilitator permit me to speak to the Master Cancer cell?" I found myself asking.

I believe that I learned to be a cancer-dancer from my four lightning strikes, from the daily not-knowing what my fate or status would be, and from the old routines and spiritual practices that are now no longer fulfilling my needs. I learned to flex-flow with the rollercoaster that has been, and will continue to be, my life.

Putting a new life pattern into place within the Integral model or any other system is difficult, as is any change of habit. Yet a cancer diagnosis can mark a turning point of intense optimism, spiritual/religious renewal, bursts of creativity, increased sensitivity, expanded compassion, and personal evolution. It is a tipping point for what might be, and a call to mobilize all that is possible within the human and divine realms.

Putting together an integral life or spiritual practice is daunting. The Integral Healing Practice calls for integrating an established Integral Life Practice (ILP)[1] with the addition of, and emphasis on, specific aspects related to health, acceptance, and flourishing. Taking the central concepts from a basic ILP and my spiritual practice accentuated my keenest and most authentic understandings of my conscious experiences, my relationships, my culture, and the systems within which I found myself.

Consciousness and Conscious Experiences

My ability to work with my cancer journey and the struggles that ensued depended heavily upon the breadth of my conscious awareness. As consciousness has already been discussed, I can summarize it as the "I/eye" that sees, and that what I can see limits or expands what I do see. Consciousness includes the ability to take others' perspectives, and begins with the clarity by which I am aware of myself. I wanted to know how "radically inclusive" I could be of all the information, emotions, and thoughts arising within me.

Dr. Baron Short, a physician who practices Integral Medicine, has argued that human awareness includes ever-increasing horizons

---

1 ILP is the practice of body, mind, and spirit in self, culture, and nature. It is the personal expression of the Integral model. ILP focuses on creating a customized approach to the quadrants, levels, lines, states, or types of one's own potential.

that are nested in what Wilber refers to as a process of "transcend and include." I have adapted Short's presentation of the layers of perception to explain how I became aware of my struggles with my illness, and thus how I envisioned myself as a cancer dancer.

Cancer dancers need to exercise their awareness of the layers of reality. When first diagnosed, there is an overlay and interplay of physical facts, cultural embeddedness (such as my familial story and mindset of victimization), emotional upheaval, and what the medical system proposes to treat the disease.

I began by exploring how any moment in time can be analyzed by looking at the simplicity or complexity of the quadrants. In addition to separating my experience into quadrants with truth claims, I also needed to be aware of the factors that hit me upon my diagnosis: the three layers of experience of Body, Mind, and Spirit, aided by the gross, subtle, and causal bodies that support them. This exercise in awareness turned muddied suffering into an object of attention, and then into an action-plan that resonated with the deepest parts of me. Seeing that the cancers were "Other" to me, and not retribution for past misdeeds or in compliance with a sad life story, alleviated the worst of my suffering. Becoming aware of how my body was registering the severity of my medical news also assisted me in grounding my emotions and preventing me from using my usual escape mechanism of dissociation.

It was quite normal that my first utterance after diagnosis was, "Am I going to die?" I was thrown back at that moment into a survival mode of thinking, even though during normal functioning I have a much higher level of cognitive awareness. Once told that I had "run-of-the-mill" breast cancer, and being given some satisfactory statistics of 10-year survival rates, I moved beyond an emergent panic over imminent death.

The maladaptive cultural functioning I learned from my family of origin was another story, and that Lower-Left influence on my behavior and emotions had to be dealt with by depth psychology and the intuitive healing provided by Lorraine. When employed by a practitioner familiar with the Integral model, depth psychology can be of great benefit in helping identify post-postmodern understandings of the ground of all being; what our original face looked like before we were born; how Christ consciousness fits in with healing; or how the *Tibetan Book of the Dead* can assist in various stages of crisis or tranquility.

Lorraine also worked methodically and intuitively to have me explore deep grief work over the disappointments and despoliations of my life. I had to become aware of old life scripts, such as "the curse of the Greenbergs," that haunted me and yet held me in their sway. I also had to confront my generalized anxiety and to come to realize that any new trauma might swing me into depression. Being confronted by an individual showing signs of borderline personality can still trigger me, but my return to normal emotional functioning is much quicker.

What I managed to do with my support staff, most of whom were not conversant with the Integral model, was to stick to reporting as accurately as possible both my subjective and my objective sensations and thoughts. I have a tendency to become verbose in both my thinking and presenting, and it was essential that I pare down my own interpretations so that I had a common language with my support team. As I learned how to simplify yet not dilute my experiences, I received wisdom from the most unlikely sources.

Honing my subjective and objective experiences into True and Beautiful statements helped me to slow down my thinking and simplify the experience. This is a similar technique to paying attention to a flame, breath, mandala, or any other object of attention. What results is a "sense of freedom and subtle, primordial feelings of peace" (Short, 2012). With support, I began to ask, "Who am I? Who is aware of these feelings, these sensations and these thoughts?" until I arrived at a sense of unbelievable spaciousness and peace.

For example, I am feeling pain on my left side where I had three surgeries and lymph nodes removed. I am aware of the pain. It is a sensation of pain, of sticking and nerves sending signals of distress right under my left arm…. It flashes off and on….Now it is not there… The phone rings and I am no longer aware of the sticking pain, but aware that I am listening to my husband change his plans for the afternoon…Where did the pain go when I was on the phone?…Gone once I was aware of something else. I was not in pain then, was I?

252

Cancer dancers are acutely aware of somatic sensations. Where is the pain? Tension? Energy? What might it imply about my overall health at this moment?

Such attentiveness is transcended and included into our original awareness. This assisted me in practices that got me deeply into my body, an area from which I am usually dissociated. I cannot do yoga for various physical reasons, but I needed to enter into bodily awareness for pain management, for the ability to report symptoms and reactions to my support team, and to permit my body to "communicate" its intelligence to me for self-healing.

Lorraine and Patricia had me do nightly body scans and to breathe into areas of tension and pain. I tensed various muscles and then focused on their relaxation. I reported many images flashing into my mind, and several of them proved supportive in my quest for psychological healing. I captured an image during meditation of what I later identified as an octahedron, or two pyramids joined at their bottoms. When I investigated this shape further, I found it was associated with the integration of the intellect, new beginnings, and mental activity—a very good portrayal of the elements at my core, I felt. By happenstance, a client had given Lorraine this very translucent crystalline shape as a gift, and she handed it to me. Now when I am overly stressed, I visualize the octahedron as rotating in my heart to give me that integration.

At the beginning of my cancer journey I was completely out of touch with my gross body and could not report much about how cold or warm I was, or where in my body I was experiencing pain. Many times I was told that I was rubbing my knee when I was unaware that it was actually throbbing with pain. The energy I learned to identify in my body then opened me up to register subtle energies that I had not previously understood.

For example, the last time I was in my sister-in-law's presence, I could have sworn she physically shoved me back with both her hands after a superficial "Hello," but I knew that such an event had not occurred. It was only later I came to understand I was experiencing her subtle energetic rage, which she could not express openly that evening. Had she actually pushed me that would have been a manifestation of gross energetic, which we all know through our waking states.

Subtle energies are also part of alternative healing modalities and may be considered part of the basic life forces of all sentient beings. Subtle energy can be identified as that which is felt during dreaming sleep and esoteric practices. Beyond the subtle state and energies are the causal and nondual (unitive). The causal is "experienced" by us all during deep, dreamless sleep while nondual states are experienced when there is no distinction between waking and dreaming, and there is no longer a distinction between experiencing ones' self as the subject or the object of a state or happening.

Another area similar to the first two is paying attention to my five senses: seeing, hearing, smelling, tasting, and touching.

My senses of smell and taste were profoundly affected as a result of chemotherapy. Oddly, for months I could not drink anything made with water; it tasted like oil. After losing 12 pounds in my first two weeks of treatment, I discovered that watermelons were a new delight, and I ate them for three meals a day until Dr. G urged me to experiment further in my quest for tolerable foods.

My next experiment unearthed the fact that I enjoyed "white" foods, from cauliflower to pasta, and for months that was my staple. The one positive relationship with food during my treatment was that dieting was not part of the treatment plan, and I was urged to consume pleasurable calories however I could come by them. My meals featured glorious delicacies and freshly made culinary efforts, which delighted my other senses and did not permit me to feel victimized by the side effects.

When my energy level waned, I cocooned myself in bed in a pair of highly prized pajamas that I felt were resort-worthy. I chose colorful silks and engaged in sensations of touch and smell in my bath and shower. When my hair began to wither and fall out, I decided to have it shaved off and invented a ritual to make it more comedic than sorrowful. My son-in-law had received some stinging criticism when we first met: he had a shaved head, and with his 6'5" frame he looked frightening to me. Later, he grew back his luxuriant hair and became a much-loved son. I gave him the "honor" of shaving my head for some karma leveling, which I felt was due for

254

past judgments. Afterward, I went shopping for a wig with a fashion-conscious friend, who helped me choose a model that so closely replicated my natural color and wave that other friends had no idea I had no hair underneath.

As for clothing post-mastectomy, there is a wonderful catalogue by the American Cancer Society entitled TLC that sells everything from wigs to scarves to prosthetic breasts. I chose several wigs and different prosthetic breasts made of a variety of materials for their feel and their look underneath my clothes. Once I felt comfortable with the fit and feel of both wig and prosthetic breast, I went on a shopping trip to Chico's for their easy-to-wear clothes. I felt chic and coddled after that retail-therapy session, and received compliments whenever I returned to Sloan-Kettering.

I made sure that I had fresh flowers and plants in my house and began to use perfume that had been collecting dust in my dressing room. Certain fragrances seemed to alter my mood dramatically, such as anything with cinnamon or heavy floral tones. I "bonded" with my houseplants, devoting the same lavish care to them as I was doing for myself. My husband teased me that the two geranium plants I rescued that fall now resembled the plant from The Little Shop of Horrors, yet my ministrations returned a sense of beauty and life to me and reminded me that regrowth and renewal were also a part of my journey.

The expensive silk pajamas I purchased for my hospital stays were a more difficult subtle exercise. I found that I constricted around the idea of splurging on myself, on this body that had been mutilated by three surgeries. When I exited the shower each day I could not help but see my missing breast and my bizarre left side, with the three deep gashes and the odd, overlapping flaps of skin left in the wake of three surgeries. I had also gained weight during chemotherapy with the prednisone I was taking, and thus I could not see anything but a bald, deformed, middle-aged woman. I first got the cheapest clothes that I could find, which in a sense was a deep reflection of how I saw my gross body.

It was only after consultations with my guides that I was able to untangle my revulsion and begin to see myself as worthy of being honored for what I had gone through. It took time, but my confused senses eventually accepted clothes that felt soft and plush.

It is natural that someone with a serious diagnosis will seek information on the Internet and in books, and the next layer of our awareness comes through feelings, thinking, and an awareness of the "self."

I have attempted to describe the range of feelings that manifested over the 18 months that I danced with cancer. It was difficult to distance myself from the incessant "monkey mind" chatter that accompanied every non-distracted waking moment. Was that ache a sign of metastatic cancer? How would this time of despair affect my immune system? What about the intense anger that I held onto from my school harassment? I found that I needed assistance in separating these thoughts from the core of what and who I was, and to appreciate them as clouds temporarily darkening a blue sky. The episode of intense bliss that I experienced at Sloan-Kettering came after I had maneuvered my sense of despair and fear out of that sky, and came to appreciate that I could and would not cease to exist in some manifestation.

I should inject a word of caution as I discuss thinking. I tend to be an inveterate researcher: newspaper articles, academic studies, websites, and books about my medical conditions quickly accumulated in my study. I read every blog and joined every breast or lung cancer listserv that I could find. It maddened me, until both my husband and Dr. G warned me to dial back the reading. As Dr. Short notes,

> Despite its gifts, we do not come genetically prepared to modulate our thinking in a modern, informational world. Given the array of digital technologies, the constant barrage—many of us are mostly living in a thought realm. A conscious state, fused and saturated with thinking, dislodges aspects of feeling, sensing... and awareness. Optimally, an individual learns to differentiate from thinking, rather than remain absorbed in the experiential stream of thoughts. (Short, 2012)

My cancers and my body's reactions to them were like no one else's, as much as I might fit into a demographic sample. To read all of the blogs and listserv comments is to receive the totality of all reactions and side effects, yet I can only react with one response that is accurate—the localized and singular me. I began to pep up once I followed their advice and stopped reading list servers and patient blogs. What I have tried to do here, with my extreme story, is to highlight a coherent practice that any person might follow regardless of how simple or complex their dance may be.

The practice of selfing, the self-dialogue practice that I have mentioned previously (not the practice of taking one's photo), allowed my voices of doom/bad luck and panicky child to have their say, but now I saw them as small slivers of who I am (i.e., a constellation of awareness, an object, and a process, all simultaneously). To reduce myself to just one of these voices would be to fall asleep to my totality.

To lessen suffering, it is important for the cancer dancer to understand the difference between what he is and what an "other" is, as well as when she is herself and not an "other." A relationship must be teased apart at all phases of the illness.

I found myself wanting to turn Dr. G and my other physicians into seers and mystics who could foretell a sunny future and protect me from evil. In psychological terms, I wanted my medical staff to be the omniscient parents who would make sure nothing bad happened to me. But I am alone in this dance with a malignant other, although my support staff can also dance with me to be of support.

We are part of an infinite system, from quarks to atoms to cells to life forms to planets and emerging solar systems. This enormous system and evolutionary context provided me with an additional layer of support. However, the cancer dancer is connected via holons (something that is both a whole in itself and a part of something larger) to something far larger than pain and uncertainty.

Integral Life Practice contains four core practice modules (Body, Mind, Spirit, and Shadow) and five supplementary ones (Ethics, Work, Relationships, Creativity, and Soul). There is also an integral spirituality practice that concentrates specifically on the core module of Spirit. There are wonderful books on integrally informed health (e.g., Dacher) and a thorough compendium on Integral Medicine (see Marilyn Schlitz).

I needed to construct an Integral Healing Practice for myself—and hopefully for others—that would support me during my many lightning strikes and move me along the continuum of coming to terms to appreciation. By adopting and adapting aspects of the practices mentioned above, I came to a healing practice that will be ongoing, since I will always have a relationship with cancer.

Recommending a practice for another requires a personal relationship between two souls: one is in crisis, and the other has been in crisis. There are so many aspects of an integral healing practice and since no one size fits all, discernment and sound judgment are required. For this reason I recommend contacting someone who can serve as an integrally informed healing mentor, be the individual a healthcare professional or an individual with personal experience in healing themselves.

I volunteer with the Cancer Hope Network, which has created a database of individuals who have experienced all types of cancers and treatment procedures. As a trained volunteer I mentor individuals who are going through precisely what I have gone through. Recently I spoke with a woman who had both breast and lung cancer and felt isolated and bizarre in having this dual diagnosis until she and I connected. I also volunteer as a cancer patient navigator with the American Cancer Society. I walk through the chemotherapy infusion suites and ask the patients if they need assistance with free wigs, makeup lessons, or managing the miseries of coming up with co-payments for their treatment. But mostly the patients want to be heard, to share their hopes and fortitude with someone who is there to listen without an agenda. I am honored to volunteer in this capacity, and to have connected with patients receptive to my cycles of healing.

There are countless cancer support groups, but not all of them will suit every individual. It is a matter of casting a wide net and seeing what is a functional fit with the individual's goals, temperament, and life conditions. But only an integrally informed healing practice can provide the cancer dancer with as complete an approach as possible in being fully supported and in being given the best opportunity to transform their lives during this liminal period.

Prior to explaining how I constructed my healing practice, it is important to note that it is not a checklist; it is a summary of all that

I examined and took as my own practice. In some cases I have listed activities or foods for general interest that are advised for people with cancer but that I did not use. I hope that what I implemented for a wide-ranging, self-constructed program might serve as guidance or inspiration for those readers affected directly or indirectly with cancer. This "emperor of all maladies" is a bitter foe and requires the broadest based attack we can muster to continue our destinies. Integral Life Practice is an excellent basis to adapt for this purpose.

The Integral Life Practice book presents full explanations of how to perform the "gold star practices" for each of the core modules. Such routines can be practiced individually or within groups created for this purpose. I need not explore this topic in more detail, as the book is readily available for interested readers. My purpose here is to add a new module on Healing.

The Self-Healing Module

Prayers for Healing

How prayer heals can be an issue for someone with no religious connection. Although I observe both Jewish and Buddhist spiritual principles, I felt the call to practice everything and anything that might help me heal, including conventional prayer.

Most often prayer is defined as a form of communion with a deity or with the Creator (Levin, 1999, p. 67). There are three basic types of prayers used by the world's wisdom traditions: 1) ritual prayer, which includes reading from a holy text or reciting memorized prayers; 2) petitionary prayer, where the supplicant requests fulfillment of spiritual or material needs such as healing; and 3) meditative prayer, where the individual quietly thinks about, worships, or listens to the Creator's voice. I hold that each form is as effective as the others and depends more on the intention of the individual praying. Rote recitations of verses taught in childhood surely are not as effective as the vulnerable pouring out of the fears and hopes of the person in need of healing. As a practitioner of integral spirituality, I am open to all denominations' prayers and styles of praying, as long as I genuinely feel comfortable doing so.

Levin proposes a theory of how these prayers might be seen as being granted and how healing might take place. The religious or practicing spiritual individual might achieve healing by virtue of his sociological environment. Many religions such as Mormonism, Judaism, and Islam observe health-related behavior such as refraining from eating certain foods, drinking, or smoking, and observing good hygiene. These practices might contribute to the epidemiologic association with increased health. During the bubonic plagues in Europe, Jews were often targeted as the causative agents of the illness for their observable absence from contracting it. We now know that it was their hygienic practices and living apart from the infected that kept them from contracting the plague. I practice what I call eco-kosher eating, which means that I select ingredients and foods that are humanely prepared and grown with an eye toward healthy living, which has been appended to the Jewish aspects of my practice. I also light Sabbath candles with my husband on Friday at sunset each week and pray in the first-, second-, and third-person for all sentient beings in need.

Second, knowing that I was the object of prayers from others must have had some healing effect since I knew that I was being supported and cared for by a large community that embraced me. In a sense, my long-held desire to be included in a community was answered in this way.

Third, Levin proposes that the knowledge that I was the object and recipient of prayers or ritualized activity (e.g., being prayed for, being on a prayer list, or having candles lit in my honor) might have stimulated my immune system. This understanding is at the core of the new field of psychoneuroimmunology (PNI), which studies the impact of feelings and emotions on the physical body. I was eternally grateful that strangers and friends thought enough about my survival that they would engage in behavior on my behalf.

Finally, there is the salutary effect of expecting healing. This harkens back to Wilber's considerations of sickness and illness. My illness was frightening indeed, particularly in light of the fact that breast cancer takes a greater toll on older women such as me, where 97% of deaths occur. But my sickness, as culturally held, might be amenable to prayer. I framed, or imbued, my cell level healing as both prayer and meditation, asking for a miraculous healing of the metastatic lymph node, and such healing did, indeed, occur. I am therefore more likely in the future to believe that such healing is possible.

Each of the categories above centered on the possible local effect of prayer on healing. But what of the marriage of prayer to quantum physics or nonlocal awareness? Unless the petitioner can hold onto a universe where disparate objects and events can be influenced instantaneously, this category of explanation would not be effective. Those who use prayer in the context of subtle energy, morphic fields, or consciousness can still hold onto a naturally ordered materialistic universe healing through nonlocal means.

How should an individual consider the possibility of supernatural mechanisms intervening to heal? I certainly faced this conundrum with my healing of the metastatic lymph node. Did the Ground of Being, the Divine, as I might name the supernatural or transcendent force in which I am subsumed, have a role in my healing? The radiologist followed the growth of my node for six months, and then on the day of the biopsy, it had simply vanished. Dr. G did not wish to analyze what had happened; she just ran over to me and hugged me joyously, twice. As a Jew, I am familiar with the concept that God operates through nature, and God also operates by supernatural miracle by violating the laws of nature. This is an example of a transcendent reality.

Levin continues his discourse on prayer by assessing its implications for healing. I received many comments from my Christian friends that my "miraculous" healing constituted "the grace of God." Cautious about slipping into a pre-rational holding of Spirit, I had to work on this concept and assure myself that I was properly attributing this healing to an at least partially transcendent Divine creator and recipient of my prayers and meditations. Where would I permit God to enter these events? My personal belief system can best be defined as panentheism, which holds that God is greater than the universe and the universe is contained within God. Thus I find that I have "room" for God in all manifestations and in all means of creation.

Affirmations for Health

Affirmations, visualization, and meditation are perfect components to a healing module. I received the following compendium from Lorraine and gathered others along the way, so I cannot state specifically what their point of origin may have been. Regardless, it is always permissible to create affirmations for specific conditions:

I am perfectly healthy in body, mind, and spirit.
I am well, I am whole, and I am strong and healthy.
I am healthy, and full of energy and vitality.
All the cells of my body are daily bathed in the perfection
   of my divine being.
I am healthy, happy, and radiant.
I radiate good health.

These affirmations to rid my body of cancer resonated intensely, and they can be made universally applicable:

I release all anger, sadness, grief, and resentment.
I lovingly forgive everyone, including myself.
I choose to fill my world with joy and peace.

Louise Hay's book, *You Can Heal Your Life,* contains an affirmation that reads more like a prayer:

In the infinity of life where I am,
all is perfect whole and complete.
I accept health as a natural state of my being.
I now consciously release any mental patterns within me
that could express as dis-ease in any way.
I love and approve of myself.
I love and approve of my body.
I feed it nourishing foods and beverages,
I exercise it in ways that are fun.
I recognize my body as a wondrous and magnificent
constellation,
and I feel privileged to live in it.
All is well in my world.

Meditation for Health

Dr. Fadel Zeidan (2010) is the lead author of a study of the effect of meditation on pain. His researchers mildly burned 15 men and women in a lab on two separate occasions, before and after the volunteers attended four 20-minute meditation-training sessions over the course of four days. During the second occasion, when the participants were instructed to meditate, they rated the exact same pain stimulus—a 120-degree heat on their calves—as being 57% less unpleasant and 40% less intense, on average.

Although this study may sound severe—and perhaps a questionable research practice—the reduction in pain ratings was substantially greater than those seen in similar studies involving placebo pills, hypnosis, and even morphine and other painkilling drugs. Zeidan reported that brain scans conducted during the pain experiments showed that this technique appeared to cause a number of changes in how the participants' brains responded to pain. Meditation reduces pain by reducing the actual sensation, Zeidan explained.

THE BODY HEALING MODULE

The list below is often recommended for physical activity for cancer patients or those in pain, and they are vital to any comprehensive healing practice:

1. Walking

This is a low-impact activity if you have the physical capability. I found it helpful that I could choose to walk in nature when called, or the mall either early with other walkers, or at any time I wanted to feel in the mainstream. During treatment I chose to walk outdoors to avoid infections.

2. Swimming

Swimming (and other forms of water exercise) defies gravity, so there aren't any unpleasant or potentially damaging jolts to the joints as I have experienced walking on asphalt.

3. Yoga

The breathing component of yoga can be just as helpful to ease chronic pain as the movement and stretching. There is chair yoga for folks such as myself that have difficulty getting down on their knees, and there are certain poses that are not recommended for postoperative patients.

4. Tai chi

Like yoga, this gentle martial art cultivates mindfulness. A New England Journal of Medicine study found that twice-weekly sessions of tai chi reduced pain, stiffness, and fatigue in fibromyalgia patients as well as helping with building strength, endurance, and balance.

5. Pilates

This increasingly popular exercise regimen helps with core strength building and can be of major benefit for anyone with low back pain or fibromyalgia. Pilates generally requires some guidance, so look for an experienced teacher.

6. Simple stretching

Anyone can do this activity in the bedroom or while waiting in line. Stretching and getting all body parts moving in a full range of motion and working just a little bit against gravity is helpful.

7. Light weight- and strength training

Weight training is particularly helpful for people suffering from arthritis, although some postoperative care instructions will caution a patient about the range of motion and weights that can be safely managed. Even lifting a can of soup can be done at home.

8. Aerobic activity

In general, aerobic activities such as using the treadmill or riding a stationary bike are particularly good for people with fibromyalgia. A meta-analysis published in the Journal of Rheumatology in 2008 found that strength-only training helped with symptoms, but that aerobic activity helped alleviate symptoms as well as improved physical function.

Food as Medicine for Health

Diet during and after cancer treatment can be a problem depending on which expert I questioned. Some studies claim that up to 50% of breast cancer cases are thought to be preventable through simple changes in diet and lifestyle.

Sloan-Kettering experts gave me a pamphlet about eating healthy, which is now being referred to as "chemoprevention." I also synthesized a list from other sources, which yielded the following foods and food-preparation tips:

Beverages
    Three cups a day of green steeped tea
    Red wine such as Pinot Noir during meals
Fruit
    Blue-, black- and raspberries
    Bananas
    Plums, peaches, nectarines
    Cherries
    Oranges, tangerines, lemons (sometime with skins grated)
    Any citrus, but organic if it has no skin
Nuts
    Walnuts, hazelnuts, and pecans
Vegetables
    Black olives without brining
    Parsley and celery
    Green vegetables and cabbage
    Carrots, yams, sweet potatoes, squash, pumpkins
    Seaweed
Seasonings, Additives
    Cold-processed extra-virgin olive oil
    Curry
    Shiitake, maitake, oyster, kawarataki, and enokitake
    mushrooms

Mint, thyme, marjoram, oregano, basil, and rosemary spices
Dark chocolate
Flaxseeds
Protein
Fish and shellfish with rich omega-3 fatty acids
Eggs
Probiotics and prebiotics
Garlic
Onions
Wheat, asparagus, or bananas
Cooking Instructions
Do not boil broccoli or other cruciferous vegetables
Do not grill, sauté, or freeze fish
Steam or slow oven-bake fresh fish

Life Extension magazine suggests adding other chemopreventive nutrients as calcium, selenium, and vitamin D3. Their November 2012 issue cites the various ways in which nutrients might fight the causative agents of breast cancer and its tendency for cells to reproduce:

By preventing DNA damage
By controlling regulatory genes
By fighting cancer-promoting inflammation
By blocking excessive cell replication
By transforming malignant cells back into healthy ones
By triggering the death of cancer cells
By restoring receptors that enhance standard breast cancer
    treatments
By inhibiting estrogen production
By blocking abnormal growth factors
By cutting off the blood supply to growing tumors
By preventing tumors from spreading

The American Cancer Society's website includes nutrition guideless for cancer prevention, for during specific treatments, and for post-treatment maintenance of good health. Dr. David Servan-Schreiber's aforementioned book, *Anti-Cancer: A New Way of Life*, contains many chapters dealing with nutrition during and after cancer treatment and is an excellent resource for coping with the appetite and digestive problems encountered during treatment.

THE CULTURAL HEALING MODULE

This module prepared me to be more patient and tolerant as I encountered medical, psychological, and spiritual specialists whom I enlisted for my support staff. This module involves connectedness at a deep level. If I stop to look around my house, I become aware of those who have made this a safe haven for me: the contractor, the furniture builders, the farmers and store owners who provided the food in my cabinets and refrigerator, my mother, laboring at her artist's easel over her lifespan to create the luscious paintings that adorn the walls, the authors who wrote the hundreds of books I have in my study, the incense maker who helped me perfume my office, and the people worldwide who designed and sewed the clothes on me and in my closet. I am aware of how each of them spoke to my values and desires.

As an individual with cancer, I have been embedded within a world of caregivers and healthcare practitioners, many of whom I have never met. Yet our interaction and relational connections permitted me to become cancer-free. I agreed to follow their culture, whether it be that of the alternative medical specialist or the maker of the chemotherapy cocktail that I consented to have infused into my body over a period of five months. I gave my utmost attention to balancing remedies in a holistic approach, which permitted a shared consciousness between the many individuals involved in my care.

Some of my caregivers did not understand either me or my values, and in these cases I needed to work on resonating with their personal or professional perspectives. For example, one of the senior hospital social workers I encountered could not make sense of my spiritual perspective. I attempted to create resonance with her perspective, but I really needed her to understand mine. No matter how earnestly I tried to explain the Integral framework, I failed to connect with her. "Oh, is your belief like the ending to The Celestine Prophecy where people ascend to another plane?" she asked in all seriousness.

My first response was scorn, but this soon softened into an I-Thou appreciation for how hard she tried to meet me, but just could not. I decided it was best not to work with her and did not join her support group. There was no mirroring, which I found to be a necessary component of those with whom I interacted and danced with. I did express appreciation for how much she cared about all of us who were afraid and suffering through our illness or treatment. The fact that I did not wish to have her join my support "staff" did not negate the spiritual compassion I felt she contained in her heart.

Each individual I encountered became an opportunity for more practice in inner development. I did not miss an opportunity to reach out to each person who came before me, and as I softened my edges, I found them coming toward me with open hearts. On the other hand, I reserved the right to be discerning about who I chose to join my support staff. I looked carefully at the list of complementary and alternative modalities and practitioners as well as the list of traditional medical modalities and practitioners and carefully deliberated which were resonant for me. It was therefore not difficult to follow the prescriptions of my chosen mixture of complementary, alternative, and traditional medicine.

THE SYSTEMS HEALING MODULE

The functional fit that I attempted to create with my support "staff" was aimed at the creation of a flowing and formless healing system. I chose the finest cancer hospital in the New York area (ranked number two in the United States). Once I had made that critical decision I had to create a map of everyone I wished to include in my healing network. The list below is an incomplete attempt to recall all who interacted with me in important ways during and after treatment:

Spouse, significant other
Nuclear family
Extended family
Close friends
Social group friends, colleagues

Teams, co-workers
Superiors, subordinates in the workplace
Pharmacists and assistants
Supermarket staff
Surgical and medical oncologists and assistants
Clinical oncologist dietician
Naturopathic oncology provider
Pain management physician
Oncologist nurses and technicians
Occupational therapist
Hospital staff
Mind-body therapist
Insurance companies
Support groups
Listserv participants
Dentists and staff
Other physicians (gynecologist, allergist, pulmonologist, cardiologist, primary care, psychiatrist)
Complementary and alternative medical practitioners (intuitive healer, homeopath)
Chemotherapy suite nurses
Friends and co-workers of spouse and family
Religious or spiritual community and leaders

This map became a healing ecology for me at the center of my being and orchestrated what I hoped might be a formless system dedicated to my healing.

Another Lightning Strike?

In September 2012, a full two years after my first lightning strike, I went to my normal group of physicians and health professionals to tell them about the events of the past two years and to have them review my non-cancer status. My immune system remained compromised for six months after the cessation of chemotherapy, and I contracted non-stop asthma and bronchial infections. I was tired of being sick and tired, so off to the pulmonologist I went.

The doctor recommended that I have a CAT scan of my remaining lung, even though I had just had one at Sloan-Kettering. His assistant called me with the alarming news that they had found a tumor on my adrenal gland. A fifth lightning strike? It felt as though I would have to return to the bald and debilitated state that I had just traversed.

After sinking into a miasma of negative thoughts, I pulled myself out long enough to contact my oncologist at Sloan-Kettering to ask whether she had seen such a tumor in my recent CAT scan. For four long hours my husband and I held our breath until the word came back that yes, they had seen a cyst, not a tumor, on this gland that is so sensitive to stress, and it was of no consequence.

Scanning the Integral map, I made a critical decision: I had to give my body-mind a full year to do deep reparative recovery work that would remove as much stress as possible. That day I wrote to the head of the seminary where I had been teaching my spiritual program and resigned. No more busy-ness. No more distress that comes from a striving human life. No more work in service of ego. No more encounters with people who do not have an interest in my surviving and thriving after my journey through cancer. I had raced back to teaching and organizational development far too quickly, so devoid of self-love and self-care was I, even after my experiences with cancer. I realized at last that there must be time invested between the phases of healing, as well as time to adapt to each new phase. I tried to gulp down appreciation and then go about my normal ways of coping with life, doing good to be appreciated by others, rather than letting the years of fear and struggle become embedded at the deepest level. I am better off than I have ever been before, and for that I weep with appreciation.

CHAPTER FIFTEEN

Conclusion

Cancer sits across the table from me. We are playing a game of unfathomable magnitude, and my very cells are the pieces that we move around the board. When Cancer first hinted a game was afoot, it teased me, it hid, it gave me false hope that I would not have to wait for hours, days, or years to know if another move was imminent. Its opening gambit was the light step of a pawn shifting forward to a neighboring square—just an ambiguous mammogram and no mass felt in my left breast. But later, when I understood the strategy, when I knew for certain my pieces—cells in my left breast and lymph nodes—had been claimed, it felt like the air collapsing just before a violent summer thunderstorm. I could not hear, I was blinded, and every nerve resonated in anguish after that first lightning strike.

In the three years since my journey began, I have sat across the desk from countless doctors and technicians for my turn to play the game. When there was good news, I would sit and smile and chat with the professional charged with helping me stay alive and cancer-free. I would then excuse myself from their office and return to my "new normal" endeavors. But when there was bad news—when Cancer decided to make a move—then I would get up from the seat and retreat once again to a place of pain and fear, planning my countermoves. After the lightning and subsequent unholy din of thunder, I pushed along the path, trying to come to terms with the new arrangement on the chess board, to adapt to this new arrangement, and then, if I was blessed, appreciate every breath until I take my last.

Both my life story and my cancer story are complex. These stories might seem unbearable to some and trivial to others; it is for this self-same reason that I offer myself and my lived experiences as a template that the reader might frame their own personal journey. My volunteer work with the Cancer Hope Network and the American Cancer Society has assured me that the phases of my journey—lightning strikes, coming to terms, adaptation, and appreciation—resonate with other cancer patients. Others have nodded their heads at my description of the mountains they scrambled up, fell down, and attempted to scramble up once again. During my own lived experience over almost three years of treatment and recovery, I found that applying the Integral model allowed me to bridge the gaps between each phase, stabilize more readily, and avoid slipping too far back during the dark periods.

The Future

I have always been a future-directed individual. I can recall the first time I read a science-fiction story at eight years old, which threw my sense of reality into a spin. It was in *Jack and Jill* magazine, and it blew my young mind open that someone could think into the unknown tomorrow and fabricate a reality. I followed this love of science fiction along with historical novels, which gave me a wide arc of literary interests. What I loved most about science and historical fiction was how reality could be molded to fix the seemingly intractable problems of modern life. Racism, poverty, war, and disease all could be navigated by bending reality and thinking along alternative lines. Writ large in both these genres is the query "What if?" which I adopted as my personal motto.

As I matured, I came to see how even small changes in my dealings with others could eventually create a sea change. This is one reason why working for three years at Integral Institute was such a dream come true for me. We theorized how an ideal integral society could form all manner of novel creations from schools to hospitals to economies. Although most of our plans did not come to fruition, they played out in how I perceive the future. And this places my daily actions within a significant context. Just as groups are fighting to awaken people to the plight of global warming and species extinction, so I, too, feel that whatever organizational or intentional moves I make must have the purpose of healing or correcting something extending into and affecting the future. This is known as evolutionary consciousness. I feel an urgency to put forward what I cobbled together over 18 months as I engaged with cancer not for my ego's sake, but for unknown yet related others who might well benefit from my story. I am a habitual sharer, of stories and of knowledge, which makes me a teacher at my core.

My Integral Healing Practice came together for me piece by piece as I read, researched, and remembered practices that I had been taught over the decades I worked with Integral Theory. As Wilber often stated, when the program comes together as a cohesive whole, something odd and spectacular happens—something he calls psychoactive (i.e., something that can only be experienced to be completely understood).

For those who believe that the Integral model is merely an anti-flatland checklist, that would be as rudimentary as believing the sun is a large glowing disc pasted against a black background. When the model is fully implemented, its dimensions expand and fill up the psyche to near bursting. More importantly, the space between lightning strikes and appreciation proceeds with little resistance, and ricocheting health pronouncements can be accommodated with understanding and grace. I was able to pace myself to make rational and heartfelt decisions about my care, and when I needed time to just be—time alone to allow the fermentation of all that I had been through—I was able to do so without looking over my shoulder and a nagging, "What if?"

The phases that I have identified do not bleed into one another seamlessly. There are fits, starts, repetitions, and plateaus, all of which I experienced during my journey—and am experiencing still. The most important quality to appreciate is that after the digestion and absorption of a lightning strike, I had to just show up for what was to occur next, not to will the next step into play. I had not experienced coming to terms while I was experiencing the multiple strikes, and thus my mandate was to pay deep attention to what was arising within me at that moment. I was also aware that I had encountered a deep mystery and thus had to wait for it to come to me. Even though I have defined the four phases of healing, I could not, and would not, want to push the moment-to-moment awareness into a false apprehension of where I "should" be in the next manifestation of my journey.

I had to experience deep faith in what was occurring within each moment. I believed that I was in touch with, and bearing witness to, something that was greater than me. Each step along the healing journey brought me into relationship with something, and when that phase ended, there was just pure mystery facing me. As a person who has had trouble trusting others, I learned to abide in a trusting relationship with something ineffable. I have rested in absolute peace more than once and am capable of reaching that clarity again.

I know that the steps along the healing journey are but mind-body reactions to that which is manifest in the gross, or material, realm. The gaps between the phases reveal the greatest mystery, which tell me that there is no mystery, only a secret: that what is real cannot change or die. I am one with the Ground of Being, and therefore, in an absolute sense, I cannot die. For the steps that I trod and continue to walk, there will be encounters with this mystery until the reality of not knowing becomes permanent and I truly have nothing to fear. Through all of the steps I have outlined, I have created an opening to learn to stand with infinity, and in that manner I expand my capacity to feel both sorrow and love.

Integral Healing Practice does not control this mystery. As with the joke about meditation, the program merely makes it more likely that I will accidentally fall into the mystery permanently. I do not delude myself into believing that I am controlling the mystery; what I am capable of controlling is the recognition that I might be falling into self-pity or victimization. I can then use the integral healing tool kit to clear my inner space so that aliveness can show up and a non-linear future will unfold before me. By non-linear I mean that instead of praying or hoping for a negative test result that will result in continued good health, I put full attention and intention toward being able to live within whatever shows up in the mystery of my true self as one with the Ground of Being.

Yet I must admit that I wish I had been able to piece my healing program together with another, be it a patient like myself or a healthcare professional on the other side of a desk. As wonderful as my providers were, as kind and caring and professional, they were not amenable to hearing more about mindfulness or meditation, and most did not encourage complementary or alternative treatment methods. So I ventured into creating a program on my own.

I know that there are other people out there who wish there were like-minded souls on the other side of the desk. This book is an attempt to locate them and to create a community that can help both healer and healee. Cancer has struck me four times, four bold moves on the board. Such is my hyper-vigilance that a missed call by a doctor who presumes there is a malignancy can send me back to feeling as though I have been struck. In the future, I hope to locate a like-minded compatriot on my medical support team so that whatever my destiny, I am accompanied by a co-healer.

I am but three years out from the first move in this unholy game. The rules, as far as I can tell, call me to evolve and thrive regardless of the severity of the strikes hurled against my body, mind, and soul. The rules are orderly: for every play sending me into searing electric pain, I must reach for appreciation for being "just so." As I go forward into not-knowing, I have several wishes. In keeping with the theme of this book, I will speak from the four perspectives of the Integral model.

Self: "I"

I have learned that all cancer patients are victims, certainly at the time of diagnosis, for this otherworldly aspect has commandeered an organ or bone or tissue that is "me" and turned it into a suicide bomber. Yet as my relationship with cancer has evolved, I realize that the "sacrifice" I have endured has been the sacrifice of ego, that of the smallness for which we mistake ourselves:

> Within the deep silence of the great unborn, Spirit whispers a sublime secret, an otherwise hidden truth of one's very essence: You, in this and every moment, abide as Spirit itself, immutable radiance beyond the mortal suffering of time and experience. Spirit itself is the very heart of one's own awareness, and it has always been so. (Wilber, 2004)

My experience of transcendent bliss and oneness with all of existence happened when I was ready to let go of all egoic tethers. I've described this numinous experience at Sloan-Kettering previously. Clad in my bathrobe alongside other bald women, the IV pole became a staff of power, the lines streaming from a bag of potions stuck into me connected me to the hearts of every other sentient being. My bathrobe was a regal cape, rustling as I strode back to my chamber. I had no opposite; there was no other, just me, smiling with fullness, inside and outside of timelessness. I remained in this brilliant transparent luminosity for months. There was nothing but love surrounding and coursing through me, embracing all the good and the bad, the pleasure and the pain I was registering yet no longer feeling in the same way. None of these dualities could touch me, yet I was ablaze with them, and I felt as though I had finally understood the Ultimate Joke, such was my joyous laughter.

I returned to my room that day transformed, cleansed, and freed from the fear of cancer or death. Pain, suffering, doubt, tears, fears, and terror had no place within me. For I saw enlightenment as a process, not as an end state, and I was in that flow which I could enter at any time by just letting go. Yet this letting go is not to be confused with despair or helplessness. Nor is it blind hope that presumes that a sunny disposition will eradicate the enemy. It calls for transcendent hope, something beyond hope that is going to fight for survival and at the same time be prepared to surrender to that which is beyond the door. In my vision I realized that the transition of death is not an "other." It is not an end to life, but rather part of a process that was ever-present and into which I fell by grace. There was no "thing" that was a polarity to life. It is this quality of pure formlessness that I pray never to forget having tasted.

Culture: "We"

I wish I could have created a sacred We-space with my medical providers. I wish that the person on the other side of the desk or the control panel were a person who might meet me with their presence and their awareness that this illness held the seeds not just of malignant growth but also transformative growth.

Many of my providers were capable of meeting my egocentric needs to alleviate suffering and my physical symptoms. They understood that my life might be shortened by the complications I faced, and they were gentle with me. How wondrous for both of us if they had lived every moment with me in sacred fullness. What a gift to all in the healing arts and those being healed if they and I had been able to create a loop of loving-kindness and appreciation for the impermanence of all life.

I considered Tom Janisse's description of levels of the doctor/patient relationship and compared it to the state of lawyer/client relationships to see where the medical establishment needs to evolve:

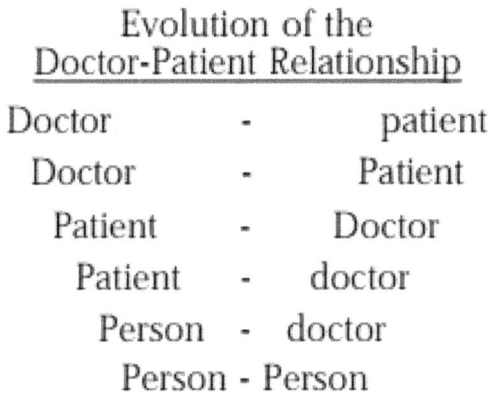

Evolution of the Doctor-Patient Relationship

Doctor	-	patient
Doctor	-	Patient
Patient	-	Doctor
Patient	-	doctor
Person	-	doctor
Person	-	Person

Figure 5. Evolution of the doctor-patient relationship.
(Janisse, 1998, p. 2).

Doctors and I, as a lawyer, have extensive postgraduate education. In the United States, attorneys are not addressed as "Doctor" as they are in some countries, although Ph.D. holders receive that courtesy. Part of this difference comes from the educational background of lawyers versus doctors. Early medical training involved apprenticeships and then moved into formal academia in separate schools with emerging standards of diagnosis and care. Attorneys apprenticed as well, but their formal movement into specialized schools occurred much later than medical professionals. Law was considered the equivalent of a bachelor's degree, and into the 1980s some states still permitted fledgling lawyers to "read" for the bar exam, meaning they could study with a private attorney without formal legal education. The law degree was formally called a "bachelor of laws," or LL.B., and it was only in the 1970s that American law schools titled their degree as Juris Doctor, or J.D.

The doctor and attorney serve patients/clients by having them come to us with their complaints. The patient arrives with bodily or psychosomatic symptoms, and the client comes to me with power imbalances. Either he is owed or owes money or rights, or he has been accused by the state or federal government of having committed a grievance against the system. In both cases, these "supplicants" believe they know what is wrong with them, and ask us both to diagnose and then treat their circumstances.

The origins of the physician can be traced back to the shaman or magical healer. The lawyer dates back to chiefs and elders. The power differential between the two, regardless of the knowledge requirements, can be seen in the quadrants they occupy. The healer deals with the Upper-Left and Upper-Right quadrants, tasked with entering and ministering to the body and the psyche. As a lawyer I am charged with the Lower-Left and Lower-Right quadrants, with the mores of culture and the rules and systems of society.

Looking at Janisse's depiction of physician/patient relationships, my medical journey began with the top row, where the doctor is in a far superior power position to the patient. This is why I addressed my doctors as "Doctor X," and they had no problem in addressing me as "Lynne." This represents the typical hierarchical relationship that remains in operation in most countries. At the height of my fear, I honestly wanted to call my surgeon Dr. Sacchini. It made me feel safe that someone in a white coat with a deferential and differentiated title would be addressing my diagnosis and illness. In contrast, my clients call me "Lynne," and I am free to call them by their first names. Consider the differential in the white coats that the doctors wear. Only in British-inspired nations do barristers wear robes and/or powdered wigs.

In Barron Lerner's *The Breast Cancer Wars*, he writes about the early days of breast cancer surgery. Patients were viewed as nothing but diseased tissue, and surgeons won praise for excising breast tissue in a series of ever more mutilating procedures. This was the opening salvo of the "war on cancer," with the surgeon as its sole hero. Lerner quotes a parody sung to the tune of "Mack the Knife" during a 1963 Christmas party about cancer surgeon George T. Pack:

278

In the morning
In the O.R.
Comes a surgeon
Big as life.
And they tell me
He needs no urgin'
For they call him
Pack the Knife.

The second level of Janisse's chart elevates the patient to one who is considered by the physician with respect, and where the medical personnel regards and treats the patient more than as just a physical machine. Many hospitals vie for the honor of receiving recognition from the likes of J.D. Power that achieve the highest levels of patient satisfaction, based on patients' perceptions and opinions:

> The J.D. Power's Distinguished Hospital Program provides hospitals with the opportunity to measure and compare patient satisfaction against established national service performance benchmarks. Hospitals that meet or exceed qualifying criteria established by J.D. Power's benchmark research are eligible for recognition as distinguished hospitals for service excellence. (J.D. Power, n.d.)

I certainly felt that I was being treated with outstanding service at Sloan-Kettering from the moment I arrived for surgeries and procedures to the time I was discharged.

I have experienced the third level with some of the medical personnel where a change occurs in the power dynamic and our relationship. Some inquired more about my personal life, dreams and fears, and listened patiently as I described my past illnesses and psychological status. I felt as though we had broken through to a partnership.

However, I have not experienced a physician who has gone beyond this evolutionary level to the "person – person" stage to ask about my psychosocial-behavioral history or my unique family story, which I believe has profound relevance to the development of my cancers. Of course, there has been sharing of life adventures and general inquiries about family members. Dr. Graham has been the kindest and most caring practitioner I have yet encountered. But patients need more: presencing, deep attention, and intentional caring.

The ideal scenario is a doctor/patient, healer/healee relationship infused with integral sensibilities and cultural awareness, so the two of us might evolve and transform together. And this is the promise of integral healing. What would cancer care look like if treatment tenets and practices were adapted in accord with Integral Theory?

I desperately wish to remain cancer-free. I have patched together the best of the four quadrants: Self, Body, Culture, and Systems. I have granted to Lorraine and Patricia equivalent status as I do my oncologists and surgeons at Sloan-Kettering. But my dream is that there will be a marriage of the healing techniques and spiritual wisdom held by my two "guides" with the skills of my traditional Western physicians. I wish that the doctors inquired about the type of psychospiritual histories that Patricia and Lorraine recorded, and that they would be able to see where or whether my early experiences possibly influenced the triggering of my two cancers. I have classified my early difficulties as a personal narrative/memoir, since I have no way to ascertain how or whether those experiences were significant factors in the cancers' development. I also wish that my doctors had been able to sit down and ask me about the healing of my metastatic lymph node.

I have done my best on my own to adapt from Eastern wisdom and Western medicine what might help me create a self-system that is as cancer-resistant as possible. U.S. culture has often distorted patients' relationship to this sickness, yet our healthcare system is barely aware of this fact. My best hope is to continue self-creating an individualized integral healing program while searching for an "other" physician who is willing to share the challenges with me.

Body: "It"

My battles with cancer and related ills are part of a "war" on a naturally occurring process within the human body. In my research on cancer, from its "discovery" in ancient Egypt, there were different truth claims about what caused it and how to eradicate it or stem its inexorable progress. Today's truth has taken us from the idea of simply amputating the sick section of the body down to looking into the cells and the DNA of the individual. After the worldwide conflicts of the 20th century we labeled our attempts to deal with cancer as a "war," with erstwhile surgeon/heroes attacking the affected body parts. These metaphors have begun to morph into "treatment" and "therapy" as we move from killing the "other" to transforming the "it."

Since scientists completed the first sequencing of a person's cancer genome in 2008, the "one size fits all" approach to cancer treatment has started to be replaced with a tailor-made treatment based on each person's DNA. Tumor profiling is coming into its own, and when I was told I might have metastatic lung cancer, I was promised a part in a clinical trial where my specific cancer profile would be targeted. These new trials will no longer consist of thousands of patients who will be followed for many years to determine if they offer minute life extensions. Indeed, the future of cancer trials will no longer be aimed at the average cancer patient. Rather, my cancer's DNA fingerprint will be tested against treatments and therapy that look for what will work just for me. Professor Alan Ashworth, Chief Executive of the Institute of Cancer Research in London, explains the effects of chemotherapy upon which I staked my very life:

> In chemotherapy for women with breast cancer, for instance, only about one in ten receives any benefit from the treatment. So that means you are massively over-treating the population—nine out of ten receive essentially no benefit. (as quoted in Connor, 2013).

Regardless of the positive statistics I was given for remaining alive if I underwent chemotherapy, my doctor was actually speaking about the average breast cancer patient and was not speaking to me personally. The "objective exterior" of cancer, which is inside me and of me, has the truth claim of scientific validity, yet "put two scientists together and you launch a truth-seeking mission" (Hawkes, 2012, p. 6). There is no "ultimate" truth, even in the objective exterior; there are only perspectives of an objective truth (i.e., there is an agreement among reputable scientists as to what constitutes a perspective on objective truth at that moment). But I will never have a personalized truth that absolutely directs me and promises me a specific result.

As we go more deeply into the body, into the "It," we are touching cells, and I have dealt with reaching them and communicating with them through cell-level meditation. This perspective will, I presume, become more widespread over the coming decades. As we come to understand the mind-body connection and the unity of the entire human within a sacred context, the more we can open up to honoring the cell as a living repository of community and communion with the larger self. And we will incorporate the cell within the mystery of our luminous energy and wisdom, emanating not just from the Divine "out there," but from and among our very cells.

What I discovered when I sat in deep meditation on those cells for a week was that I could trust my body to regain its balance. It was that presencing, intention, creative and dynamic balancing and resilience upon which I put my faith during that week. I connected with vibrancy and energy among my cells in that invaded lymph node. Like a cut clotting and the skin stitching together, I understood that the affected cells would reorganize and the cancer cells would disperse. I will forever be grateful for that experience, knowing that I am capable of it, but I am also respectful of the cells and their patterning, their communicating, their dying and birthing, and accept that I may not be able to repeat this miracle. But I know its scent, its energy, its feel.

Systems: "Its"

My hope for the future for all cancer patients begins at the moment in Dr. Woodward's office when she told me "You have invasive breast cancer," on October 1, 2010, with a dark tone and a deadpan expression. She continued, "Lynne, you have run-of-the-mill breast cancer. Just like 80% of women with cancer." I don't know if this was true, and even if it were statistically valid, I now understand that my survival rate isn't affected by the fact that I am in a cohort of 80%. I now understand that my life expectancy and my chances of metastatic cancer from either breast or lung are truly untethered from any of the statistics I have clung to over the past three years.

More importantly, I have experienced firsthand how the medical system deals with patients such as me, and I would hope that laws and healthcare ecologies associated with cancer care change dramatically. After Dr. Woodward sat with me and quickly explained the nature of my breast cancer and the possible protocols for treatment, I was then sent to the parking lot to drive home in a state of confusion, terror, and lack of focus. This is a cruel way for anyone to face a serious illness requiring invasive surgery and difficult therapy.

Integral Healing Practice can include a more comprehensive and humane method of assisting patients with a four-quadrant approach. I have been trained as a cancer patient navigator under the auspices of the American Cancer Society. In some hospitals, patient coordinators are called upon to explain terminology and medical procedures, instruct patients how to use home healthcare products, or even collect data for further research. Other hospitals literally walk the patient from the room where they have been diagnosed to a private room where coordinators and medical staff answer their immediate questions, and begin the process of bridging them from lightning strike to coming to terms. There are also hospitals such as the John Theurer Cancer Center in New Jersey that do not permit cancer patients to be without a staff member/coordinator at any time while in the hospital or while undergoing treatment.

As a patient navigator, I am forbidden by the rules to discuss spirituality or religion; I understand this, given the fact that a person must be trained to handle such a delicate subject at an extraordinarily vulnerable time. There is currently a prohibition on chaplains serving in hospitals unless they are affiliated with traditional faith traditions. Those who label themselves as interfaith, interspiritual, or integral are not permitted access to patients either in public or military hospitals. But this prohibition may well be extinguished in the coming decade as more people drift from the traditional faiths into alternative practices.

With the growing interest in spiritual and religious influence on health outcomes, I would hope that medical personnel or specially trained patient coordinators will address patients' spiritual needs when they ask about patients' needs at the moment. In the May/June 2013 issue of *Explore*, it was noted that patients saw the role of spirituality in medical encounters as closely tied to the interpersonal relationship and the psychosocial care provided by physicians. Moreover, "spiritual distress experienced by cancer patients may be under-addressed due to lack of confidence in effectiveness, and role uncertainty" (Lucchetti et al. 2013, p. 159). How might we resolve this lack of attention? I already had one spiritual advisor and obtained a second right after my diagnosis, so I was basically surrounded with loving and supportive spiritual adepts. But what of the person who cannot go to a spiritual mentor or elder, not being part of a congregation? As a first step, I would hope that medical personnel assign roles for specialists to take spiritual histories along with medical ones.

The goals of taking a spiritual history are conceived by the authors of the *Explore* article as follows:

> Share and learn about the patient's spiritual and religious beliefs
> Assess spiritual distress or strength
> Provide compassionate care
> Help the patient to find inner resources of healing and acceptance
> Identify spiritual/religious beliefs that affect the patient's treatment
> Identify those in need for referral to a chaplain or spiritual care provider

As I attended various support groups for people with cancer, it became obvious to me that right beneath the veneer of small talk about daily challenges was the explosive challenge of addressing spiritual questions, yet I never encountered any social worker or facilitator who permitted these questions to emerge. I realize that I was never part of an end-of-life support group where such questions naturally must be handled, but there is every reason for them to be permitted at whatever early or intermediate stage the cancer patient might be diagnosed. We need chaplains, companions, spiritual "buddies" or mentors, who can sit in the hospital and meet patients wherever they may be in the development of their spiritual line. That is true respect for a mind/body/soul connection that would promote integral healing.

A culture that cares about the feelings, emotions, mind-body connection of cancer patients, and all patients facing a critical illness, would not permit patients to struggle alone from the first notification of their future struggles through either the end of treatment or the notification of terminal illness. My prayer is for the medical establishment to create systems that envelop a cancer patient with caring companionship so that this solo struggle receives the support of the many.

❧

This voyage began in 2010 with my breast cancer diagnosis, flashed back to my birth in 1945, and shot forward to that fateful moment in Dr. Woodward's office. It then followed me to the present and into the future. But my story hinges on feelings of stress and how the disturbing events in my life might have contributed to my health challenges. Whether there is a direct scientific correlation between all that transpired in my life or not, this belief of mine has stood determinedly yet flexibly, depending on which perspective I choose to adopt.

From an integral perspective, no quadrant affects the totality of the individual alone; they tetra-arise and interconnect seamlessly, as did my worries. From rules that shaped the culture of my high school to the point that I fell afoul of the administration, to feeling scapegoated and fearful for my job, which led to a retinal bleed and the collapse of my immune system—all four quadrants worked together to produce my outcomes. To this run around the quadrants of Self/"I," Body/"It," Culture/"We," and Systems/"Its," I see how this quadrant was perhaps more distorted than the others. As a child, I was enmeshed in my mother's mental illness and an environment that called for me to please her lest I not be loved, which created fear and a challenged immune system. Adding to this vulnerability was my father's chain smoking and my mother's and aunt's histories of breast cancer, which impinged on my genetic and environmental worlds. The Integral model has taught me to acknowledge complexity within complexity, and I have the utmost respect for the uselessness of pointing to a single core reason for my cancers. In truth, the reasons are unknowable.

Life continued on after treatment. In my understandable quest to feel as vibrant as I had before my surgeries and chemotherapy, I pitched in to teach the spiritual program that had limped on. My mind might have been anxious to return to my prior energetic commitment, but my body was not. I was once again not in alignment with my "new normal." I had pushed myself in the spring and fall of 2012 far beyond what my body was ready to accept. I got sick with asthma and bronchitis multiple times because my immune system failed to re-ignite quickly. I lay in bed for days at a time exhausted from simple chores. Illness led to the cancellation of a post-cancer European adventure. My husband had serious back surgery after months of unrelenting pain in December and I was put back into the role of caregiver rather than self-care. Life continued to happen.

So what did I learn from cancer and why am I able to appreciate life with all of its vicissitudes far more now than before? I have learned that even at the mouth of death I am supported by Spirit. Even faced with terrible pain and trembling with fear, I can negotiate any situation and move forward. Even if the next scan shows something I'd rather turn away from, I know that I will be able to deal with its implications, and I will be able to look outside at my dogwood trees, my lilac and gardenia bushes, my cardinals and blue jays feeding at their stations, the fox that creeps around the house, the flock of wild turkeys that parade their young through our yard, and appreciate life. I will feel the soft touch of Adam's little fingers, when he throws himself on me in loving abandon, his thick blond hair and tiny toes as he crawls all over me, and know that I can appreciate the joy he represents. I smile at the still-awkward attempts of my longtime husband to show his love for me. I register the effect I have had on growing my child into a stunning and talented woman. I watch Melissa as she loves her own daughter.

I have lived through a tumultuous period of history and survived a wild and unhealthy upbringing. Yet this ultimate unhealthy time of cancer and infection seemed to permit a purging and cleansing of what kept me from living freely and more abundantly. Of course I owe so much of this to my doctors and medical assistants, to Lorraine and Patricia, and to brilliant and insightful friends such as Robin, whose companionship carried me through my "dark night of the soul."

And thus, after recounting the difficult life I have led and the lessons about appreciation, gratefulness, and love that I have learned, I, as so many before me, am left with the Mystery to uplift and support me.

A Meditation on This Moment

Shehecheyanu

Shehecheyanu, v'kiy'manu, v'higianu laz'man hazeh.

O Mystery, Grace unfolding, O miracle, it's You alone,

O Mystery, Grace unfolding, O Miracle, who brings us Home.

– Rabbi Shefa Gold

References

American Cancer Society. (2011). Attitudes and cancer. Retrieved June 30, 2013, from http://www.cancer.org/treatment/treatmentsandsideeffects/emotionalsideeffects/attitudes-and-cancer.

Arun, B., Dunn, B.K., Ford, L.G., & Ryan, A. (2010). Breast cancer prevention trials. *Seminars in Oncology, 37*(4), 367-383.

Bernhard, T. (2010). *How To Be Sick: A Buddhist-Inspired Guide for the Chronically Ill and Their Caregivers.* Boston, MA: Wisdom Publications.

Brodsky, J. (1986). *Less Than One: Selected Essays.* New York: Farrar Straus Giroux.

Chodron, P. (1996). *When Things Fall Apart: Heart Advice for Difficult Times.* Boston, MA: Shambhala.

Chodron, P. (2003). *Comfortable With Uncertainty: 108 Teachings on Cultivating Fearlessness and* Compassion. Boston, MA: Shambhala.

Choi, K-E., Rampp, T., Saha, F.J., Dobos, G.J., & Musial, F. (2011). Pain modulation by meditation and electroacupuncture in experimental Submaximum Effort Tourniquet Technique (SETT). *EXPLORE: The Journal of Science and Healing, 7*(4), 239-245.

Cohen, A. (2012). *Enough Already: The Power of Radical Contentment.* Carlsbad, CA: Hay House.

Connor, S. (2013, January 28). Forensic cancer treatment: Personalised drug therapy becoming a reality with hopes for improvement in survival rates. *The Independent.*

Coyne, J.C., & Tennen, H. (2010). Positive psychology in cancer care: Bad science, exaggerated claims, and unproven medicine. *Annals of Behavioral Medicine, 39*(1), 16-26.

Dacher, E. (2006). *Integral Health: The Path to Human Flourishing.* Laguna Beach, CA: Basic HealthPublications.

Dacher, E. (2011). *Aware, Awake, Alive: A contemporary Guide to the Ancient Science of Integral Health and Human Flourishing*. St. Louis, MO: Paragon House.

deMello, A. (1990). *Awareness: The Perils and Opportunities of Reality*. New York: Doubleday.

Dossey, L. (2006). *The Extraordinary healing Power of Ordinary Things*. New York: Harmony Books.

Douglas, T. (1995). *Scapegoats: Transferring Blame*. Milton Park: Routledge.

Ehrenreich, B. (2009). *Bright-Sided: How Positive Thinking is Undermining America* New York: Henry Holt and Company.

Freeman, S. (n.d.) How the placebo effect works. Retrieved August 1, 2013, from http://health.howstuffworks.com/medicine/medication/placebo-effect1.htm.

Esbjörn-Hargens, S. (2012). An overview of Integral Theory: An all-inclusive framework for the 21st century.

Gold, *The Magic of Hebrew Chant*.

Grof, S., & Grof, C. (Eds.). (1989). *Spiritual Emergency: When Personal Transformation Becomes a Crisis*. New York: Putnam.

Hafiz. (1999). *The Gift: Poems by Hafiz*. Ladinsky, D. (Trans.). New York: Penguin Group.

Hahn, T.N. (2003). *No Death, No Fear*. New York: Riverhead.

Harris, A.H, Luskin, F.M., Benisovich, S.V., Standard, S., Bruning, J., Evans, S., & Thoresen, C. (2006). Effects of a group forgiveness intervention on forgiveness, perceived stress and trait anger: A randomized trial. *Journal of Clinical Psychology*, *62*(6), 715-733.

Hawkes, J.W. (2012). *Resonance: Nine Practices for Harmonious Health and Vitality*. New York: Hay House.

Hay, L. (1984). *You can Heal Your Life*. Carlsbad, CA: Hay House.

Helminski, K. (Ed.). (1998). *The Rumi Collection*. Boston, MA: Shambhala.

Heszler, P. (n.d.). Hope as irrational, immanent, and transcendent. Retrieved August 1, 2013, from http://www.crvp.org/book/Series03/IIIB-10/chapter-7.htm.

Holistic Integrative Therapies. (n.d.). Homepage. Retrieved July 11, 2010, from http://www.holisticintegrativetherapies.net/.

Janisse, T. (1998). Editor's comments. *The Permanente Journal, 2*(3), 2-3.

J.D. Power. (n.d.). The distinguished hospital program. Retrieved August 1, 2013, from http://www.jdpower.com/business-services/services/certification/distinguished-hospital-program.htm.

Johnson, A. (2012, November). Epigenetics: for breast cancer prevention. *LifeExtension*. Retrieved August 21, 2013, from http://www.lef.org/magazine/mag2012/nov2012_Epigenetics_Breast_Cancer_01.htm.

Kay, P., Grundland, B (2009). *Cell Level Meditation.* Olympia, WA: Simply Wonder.

Lerner, B.H. (2003). *The Breast Cancer Wars: Hope, Fear, and the Pursuit of a Cure in Twentieth-Century America.* New York: Oxford University Press.

Lesser, E. (2004). *Broken Open: How Difficult Times Can Help Us Grow.* New York: Villard.

Levin, J. (1999). *Essentials of Complementary and Alternative Therapies.* Philadelphia, PA: Lippincott Williams & Wilkins.

Levin, J. (2001). *God, Faith, and Health: Exploring the Spirituality-Healing Connection.* New York: John Wiley and Sons, Inc.

Lucchetti, G. Bassi, R.M., & Granero Lucchetti, A.L. (2013). Taking spiritual history in clinical practice: A systematic review of instruments. *Explore: The Journal of Science and Healing, 9*(3), 159-170.

Maitri, S. (2000). *The Spiritual Dimension of the Enneagram: Nine Faces of the Soul.* Los Angeles, CA: Tarcher.

Martinez, M. (2009). *The mind-body code* [audio interview]. Boulder, CO: Sounds True, Inc.

Mathews, A. (2007). *Restoring My Soul: A Workbook for Finding and Living the Authentic Self.* Bloomington, IN: iUniverse.

Mayo Clinic. (n.d.). Cancer treatment myths: Any truth to these common beliefs? Retrieved January 7, 2013, from www.mayoclinic.com/health/cancer/HO00033/NSECTION-GROUP=2.

McBride, K. (2008). *Will I Ever Be Good Enough?* New York: Free Press.

McNerney, A. (2004). *The Gift of Cancer: A Call to Awakening* Baltimore, MD: Resonant Publishing.

Memorial Sloan-Kettering Cancer Center. (2011). *Nutrition and Breast Cancer: Making Healthy Diet Decisions.* New York: Memorial Sloan-Kettering Cancer Center.

Mukherjee, S. (2010). *The Emperor of All Maladies.* New York: Scribner.

Namka, L. (n.d.). Scapegoating: An insidious family pattern of blame and shame on one family member. Retrieved July 1, 2012, from http://www.byregion.net/articles-healers/Scapegoating.html.

Online Etymology Dictionary. (n.d.). Victim. Retrieved August 26, 2012, from http://dictonary.refeence.com/.

Orenstein, P. (2013, April 28). Our feel-good war on breast cancer. *New York Times Magazine.*

Orloff, J. (2011). The power of an animal's unconditional love. *Psychology Today.* Retrieved February 13, 2013, from http://www.psychologytoday.com/blog/emotional-freedom/201111/the-power-animals-unconditional-love.

Palmer, P. (2011). *Healing the Heart of Democracy: The Courage to Create a Politics Worthy of the Human Spirit.* San Francisco, CA: Jossey-Bass.

Parlee, B. (2010). Integral optimism: How to face our epic global challenges with informed hope and faith. Fall|Winter, *Kosmos Journal.*

Post, S., & Niemark, J. (2007). *Why Good Things Happen to Good People: The Exciting New Research That Proves the Link Between Doing Good and Living a Longer, Healthier, Happier Life.* New York: Broadway Books.

Preece, R. (2006). *The Wisdom of Imperfection.* Boulder, CO: Snow Lion Publications.

Rabin, R.C. (2011). A pink-ribbon race, years long. Retrieved August 1, 2013 from http://www.nytimes.com/2011/01/18/health/18cancer.html?pagewanted=all.

Richardson, P.T. (1996). *Four Spiritualities: Expressions of Self, Expressions of Spirit*. Palo Alto, CA: Davies-Black Publishing.

Richmond, L. (2012). *Aging as a Spiritual Practice*. London: Gotham Books.

Rinpoche, C.T. (1992). *Transcending Madness: The Experience of the Six Bardos*. Boston, MA: Shambhala.

Rinpoche, S. (1994). *The Tibetan Book of Living and Dying*. San Francisco, CA: Harper.

Riso, D. (1990). *Understanding the Enneagram: The Practical Guide to Personality Types*. Boston, MA: Houghton Mifflin Company.

Riso, D., and Hudson, R. (1999). *The Wisdom of the Enneagram: The Complete Guide to Psychological and Spiritual Growth for the Nine Personality Types*. New York: Bantam Books.

Salzburg, S. (2003). *Faith: Trusting Your Own Deepest Experience*. New York: Riverhead.

Schlitz, M. (2005). *Consciousness and Healing: Integral Approaches to Mind-Body Medicine*. St. Louis, MO: Elsevier.

Servan-Schreiber, D. (2009). *Anti Cancer: A New Way of Life*. New York: Viking.

Short, B. (2012). Advancing integral perspectives in psychiatry: Part 1. *Journal of Integral Theory and Practice*, 6(4), 41-56.

Simonton, O.C., Matthews-Simonton, S., & Creighton, J.L. (1978). *Getting Well Again*. New York: Bantam Books.

"Soul Progress." Self-transcendence. Retrieved December 15, 2012, from http://www.soulprogress.com/html/Glossary/Self-TranscendenceGlossary.html

Sulik, G. (2012). *Pink Ribbon Blues: How Breast Cancer Culture Undermines Women's Health*. Oxford: Oxford University Press.

Taylor, T. (2008). *A Spirituality for Brokenness: Discovering Your Deepest Self in Difficult Times*. Woodstock, VT: Skylight Paths Publishing.

Thermography Clinic, Inc. (n.d.). Carcinogenic personality profile. Retrieved August 11, 2012, from http://www.drmostovoy.com/carcinogenic_personality_profile.htm.

Tolomeo, D., Gervais, P., & De Roo, R.J. (2001). *Biblical Characters and the Enneagram*. Victoria: Newport Bay Publishing.

Verhoef, M.J., & Mulkins, A. (2012). The healing experience—how can we capture it? *EXPLORE: The Journal of Science and Healing, 8*(4), 231-236.

Walsh, R., & Shapiro, S. (2006). The meeting of meditative disciplines and western psychology: A mutually enriching dialogue. *American Psychologist, 61*, 227-239.

Weil, A. (2004). *Health and Healing: The Philosophy of Integrative Medicine and Optimum Health*. New York: Mariner Books.

Wilber, K. (1996). *The Atman Project: A Transpersonal View of Human Development* [second edition]. Wheaton, IL: Quest Books.

Wilber, K. (1998). *The Essential Ken Wilber: An Introductory Reader*. Boston, MA: Shambhala.

Wilber, K. (2000). *One Taste: Daily Reflections on Integral Spirituality*. Boston, MA: Shambhala.

Wilber, K. (2001). *Grace and Grit: Spirituality and Healing in the Life and Death of Treya* Killam Wilber [second edition]. Boston, MA: Shambhala.

Wilber, K. (2004). *The Simple Feeling of Being: Embracing Your True Nature*. Boston, MA: Shambhala.

Wilber, K. (2007). *Integral Spirituality: A Startling New Role for Religion in the Modern and Postmodern World*. Boston, MA: Shambhala.

Wilber, K., Patten, T., Leonard, A., & Morelli, M. (2008). Integral Life Practice: A 21st-Century *Blueprint for Physical Health, Emotional Balance, Mental Clarity, and Spiritual Awakening*. Boston, MA: Integral Books.

Yoder, J.H. (1971). *The original revolution: Essays on Christian pacifism*. Harrisonburg, VA: MennoMedia.

Zeidan, F., Gordon, N.S., Merchant, J., & Goolkasian, P. (2010). The effects of brief mindfulness meditation training on experimentally induced pain. *Journal of Pain, 11*(3), 199-209.

Zeidan, F., Martucci, K.T., Kraft, R.A., Gordon, N.S., McHaffie, J.G., Coghill, R.C. (2011). Brain mechanisms supporting the modulation of pain by mindfulness meditation. *Journal of Neuroscience, 31*(14), 5540-5548.